A...
Christians Can Like It Too

A Complete Guide To Anal Play Without Pain

Kelly Walls

Table of Contents

You Will Learn in This Book

Other Books By Kelly Walls

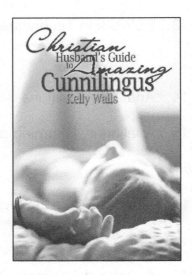

Are you giving your wife screaming orgasms?

If not you're like most guys that have no idea how to stimulate the clitoris. Is your wife shooting you in the face with so much cum you feel like you need goggles? Don't you dare settle for the lie that she is not a squirter! All women can squirt if they're stimulated correctly. So many men don't have a clue how to stimulate the clitoris. They finally find it and say to themselves; "there it is I guess I should rub it real hard." "WRONG!"

My friend there is a reason why it is protected by a hood and most of it is hidden except for the tip. It is because its only purpose is for her sexual pleasure. If you apply the principles in this book your wife will squirt you most of the time. She will scream with pleasure. She will wiggle all over the bed and grab your head and push it into her pussy and scream and call you a SEX God!

Listen to me guys, eating your wife's pussy is about the most wonderful thing you can do for her. It makes her feel specially loved, admired, sexy, and of course it makes her cum like crazy. In fact, statistics prove that many women prefer it to intercourse, and for most women it is the easiest way to cum with her man.

You may have the smallest penis on the planet, but if you give great cunnilingus, you will be appreciated as a fabulous lover. Yes, it's that important. Besides, lots of women expect it these days. So, you might as well know what you're doing.

Fellas, if you don't know it by now, know this. Cunnilingus is amazing to women! And all men must learn to respect the clitoris of their wife. It's a sex organ given to them by God Himself for only one function alone and that is to bring her pleasure. And with its more than 8,000 nerve endings, it does just that!

The main problem is that many men are reluctant to give their wife cunnilingus. Either they don't like to do it, they don't know how to do it, they don't do it often enough, or they don't do it long enough when they do-do it.

And worst yet of the guys that do give cunnilingus, not all of them know how to do it well. And most of them don't know how to set their wife at ease so she enjoys the experience to the fullest. Christian friends this book is your answer with more than 210 cunnilingus tips alone, you are sure to find something that will send your wife over the edge.

This book has been called the encyclopedia of the art of cunnilingus filled to the brim with over 100 pages of pure teaching on giving cunnilingus, vaginal and anal massaging, rimming and so much more. And if that was not enough more practice will give you a deeper understanding of the practice and help you and your honey have a better oral experience together.

And of course, as with all our books it is written from a Christian perspective taking into consideration what God has to say or has not to say about various topics. This I believe will help you take your cunnilingus skills to a new level.

Consider this sad fact guys. The average man who practices coital relations, that is thrusting into his wife's vagina lasts approximately 2 and a half to three minutes and the average woman take approximately fifteen to twenty minutes to reach her first orgasm.

So, what you do in the first twelve and a half minutes really makes the difference as to whether she will experience true pleasure at all. I fear that most woman end up finishing themselves off with their fingers after their husband is sleeping. This shouldn't be so in a vibrant healthy marriage. And most woman if they will admit it to you enjoy cunnilingus more that penetration from a penis.

Personally, I don't care if I get my wife off with my tongue, finger or penis as long as I get the job done and she enjoys the intimacy. As long as I leave her breathing hard and begging me to stop because she can't take it anymore, then I am pleased.

This book will teach you how to give her multiple orgasms with both your tongue and your fingers, also if you want a more detained guide on fingering and pleasing your wife with your hands get my book "Christian Husbands Guide to Fingering and Pleasuring His Wife with his Hands." When you leave the bedroom, you will know that you pleased her and she will want to pleasure you with better fellatio too.

My friend most women want to reciprocate pleasure so you can get her my Fellatio book; "Christian Wife's Guide To Pleasuring Her Husband With Great Fellatio" for present and give it to her. It has over 200 fellatio techniques in it. **Get a copy today!**

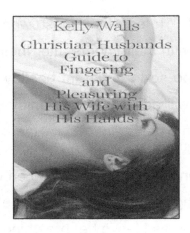

Is your wife screaming and squirting and begging you to stop because she can't take another orgasm? If not, maybe the problem is you don't know how to use your fingers. You see sir the G spot is the pleasure center for the woman. And he clit was given to her by God for the sole purpose of orgasm. And to make matters worse most guys don't know how to touch it properly. They don't know how to stimulate it correctly. Most guys just sort of poke and rub all around hoping they do something that she likes. **If she isn't asking you to use your fingers on her then you don't know what you're doing!**

Another interesting fact is that most guys penises are shaped to stimulate the G spot, but they don't how to do it with them. Some men think they have to have a 10-inch penis to pleasure their wife. Not so my friend. I can show you how to do it and make her beg you for it with just your thumb. In fact, my wife prefers a thumb ride as she playfully calls it over any other kind of way to pleasure her sexually.

I'll show you how to make circles with your fingers that will make her squirt and scream at the same time. You will learn dozens of finger techniques to masturbate your wife with and stimulate her G spot with. I promise if you use these techniques rubbed against the G-spot you will cause her to squirt at least half the time. She will go wild in bed and want to pleasure you as well. You might want to get her my new hand job secrets book that's filled with masturbation techniques that she can use on you to pleasure you as well. And believe me she wants to pleasure you.

The techniques you will learn will make you have to put a towel on your bed before you make love to her with your fingers. Okay gents you want to learn more about pleasuring your wife with your hands that's why you are buying this book.

This book is a definitive guide to the female vagina and inside this guide you'll learn...

- step-by-step, techniques on how to finger your wife the proper way that will give her a mind-blowing orgasm.
- How to stroke her clitoris to produce clitoral orgasms and multiple orgasms are usually common.

- How to combine oral sex and fingering techniques.
- The best positions to finger your wife in during sex that will make her reach climax every time and not just about 40% of the time.
- Step-by-step instructions on how to find the G-Spot and what to do once you find it. Even how to play with her anus if she wants you too.

Guys this is the key to making her squirt you in the face with a squirting orgasm. Even if she has never squirted before these techniques will teach her how to get her to squirt with pleasure.

Anal fingering and massaging and the amazing pleasure that comes from this practice.

Dozens of techniques and strategies that will lead your wife to orgasmic bliss. A great buy! **So, get a copy today and have some fun! Buy a copy now!**

Chapter 1

Is Anal Sex A Sin For Christian Couples?

All married Christian couples eventually come to "that topic:" that is the big question we all need an answer to, is anal sex a sin in a Christian marriage? Is anal sex okay for the married Christian couple to partake in sexuality for their own pleasure? Many churches have adamantly condemned anal sex as being a sin calling it sodomy which is a sin, but why? Does the bible say that it is a sin for heterosexual couples to have anal sex with each other?

No, the Bible does not say that anal sex is a sin for married Christian couples or any married opposite sex couples for that matter. Despite Old Testament purity laws regarding women's periods, there are no limitations put on anal sex as a part of Christian sexuality in a marriage. Some try to say that anal sex is sodomy, and it is a sin for two men to participate in. Yes, two same sex men having anal sex is a sin. But so is two men kissing passionately or same sex couples getting married. Sodomy is not anal sex between and husband and wife.

So, if it is not blatantly a sin, is anal sex okay in a Christian marriage?

Maybe?

Let us first consider how it might be wrong for a couple to participate in it. If a husband demands that his wife engage in anal sex, and she is not comfortable with it, that intentionally violates the trust in the sexuality of a Christian marriage. ANY sexual practice that both partners are not comfortable with is wrong, not biblically, but morally between that couple.

Now, let's also consider how anal sex may be an okay addition to the sexuality in a Christian marriage. If both partners desire anal sex, it may be okay for them. If both partners understand the risks of anal sex in a marriage, then it may also be okay for them. If neither partner feels degraded by the sex act, it may be okay for them.

Here is a checklist to determine if it is OKAY

Do we feel anal sex is a sin in a Christian marriage?

Are we both emotionally prepared for anal sex in our marriage? Do we really understand the risks and precautions that we must take when adding anal sex to our Christian marriage sexuality? In today's loose modern day anal play has become a popular thing in many marriages, even in Christian marriages. And always remember that you don't have to have full-blown anal sex to enjoy some fun back door play. Anal play includes many things. He or she can lube up a finger and use it to caress you either around that area or directly in the anus itself.

There are many nerve endings located there, so it's understandable that both men and women can get some wonderful sensations from caressing that area. This type of FUN FINGER PLAY can also be used to heighten oral sex and regular intercourse as well.

Ladies If you are curious as to whether or not you would enjoy this experience my advice to you is, the next time you are on top of your husband during cowgirl sex, ask him if he'd reach around and caress your butthole back there. If he wants to, he can wear a latex glove. Or, even the next time when you are masturbating, caress yourself back there, and see how it feels to you. If you like it, and it feels erotic to you, then you could also try inserting a lubed finger and see what kind of sensations that gives you.

Okay say you like the feeling and you have decided to give it a try, so what are some pointers? You've bought the right book for that's what this book is about. A book filled with pointers to help you get started on the right path and not do so with guilt and condemnation. Still not convinced it's okay in a Christian marriage? Now before we go any further let's look at some scriptures and see what the bible has to say about the just of anal sex.

Chapter 2

Anal Sex, What Does the Bible Say?

The bible carefully spells out many sins for us. God's word tells us that adultery is a sin. It is even a commandment not to commit it.

Leviticus 18:20 (King James Version) 20 *Moreover thou shalt not lie carnally with thy neighbor's wife, to defile thyself with her.*

Exodus 20 (King James Version) *And God spake all these words, saying,* 14 *Thou shalt not commit adultery.*

His word also tells us fornication and bestiality are sins. Fornication is simply defined as unlicensed sexual behavior. So, for those of you that say marriage is just a piece of paper, Sorry! Bestiality, well that is self-explanatory.

1 Corinthians chapter 6:18 (King James Version) 18 *Flee fornication. Every sin that a man doeth is without the body; but he that committeth fornication sinneth against his own body.*

1 Thessalonians Chapter 4:3 (King James Version) 3 *For this is the will of God, even your sanctification that ye should abstain from fornication:*

1 Corinthians Chapter 7:2 (King James Version) 2 *Nevertheless, to avoid fornication, let every man have his own wife, and let every woman have her own husband.*

Leviticus chapter 20:15-16 (King James Version) 15 *And if a man lie with a beast, he shall surely be put to death: and ye shall slay the beast.* 16 *And if a woman approach unto any beast, and lie down thereto, thou shalt kill the woman, and the beast: they shall surely be put to death; their blood shall be upon them.*

In case you may be wondering the bible doesn't, spell it out any specifics for heterosexual anal sex. There are no specific verses that say that anal sex between married couples is a sin. There are verses that TALK ABOUT homosexuality, but not a married couple. I believe that if it were a sin, God would have included it in with the others he mentioned. But since the bible is totally silent on this issue, there is an ongoing debate among well-meaning Christians regarding this practice in a marriage.

This is something that you and your spouse will need to discuss together in private and pray about. The Holy Spirit will convict you as to what is best for your marriage. If one of you has a history of deep porn addiction before Christ, where anal sex was depicted and highlighted in the wrong mode, then it's possible that engaging in anal sex could become a slippery slope for you, and lead you back into your old, sinful lifestyle choices. You'll need to ask yourself: *Will doing this cause me to lust for more sex or for sex with others? Will it remind me of the pornography and cause me to revert back to that?* While participating in anal sex may be okay for one couple, it may cause another couple to stumble.

This is really important my friend. Just because something is completely and totally permissible, that does not necessarily mean that it's beneficial to you. There are precautions and health concerns that you need to be aware of before you get active in anal play. Cleanliness is important, and so is being gentle and taking it slow at first.   Some couples may be interested in anal sex or anal play, but after weighing all the pros and cons, decide that it isn't edifying for their marriage. I respect and understand this. I humbly ask for that same respect in the decisions that my wife and I have made. My prayer for you is may, God bless your marriage and your individual decisions! I feel you want to know more about it so you can make a conscience decision that's why you purchased this book. So I will endeavor to give you a lot of information on how to practice, safe, enjoyable God glorifying anal sex. (*And guys it isn't always sticking your penis in and pounding her for all you are worth.*) As I've already stated anal sex isn't for everyone, but it can be interesting to try if you don't have many inhibitions and you're happy to experiment sexually and have fun.

Well, to start things off, if you and your spouse have decided to try some anal play, please make sure that their fingernails are trimmed nice and short. Trust me on that one. My wife hates any small snags, so I know for sure what I'm saying. You will have to use some extra lube for the anus makes none of its own. We like ID Glide or Astroglide or you can use coconut oil if you want to try analingus because it is tasteless… More on that later.

A lubed finger feels so much better down there. Make sure that you shower or bathe beforehand and are really clean. That needs no explanation. (I hope) Remember to never re-insert anything back into the vagina, after it has been in the rectum. And finally, if you aren't sure about incorporating this into your sex life, or if you are just shy about trying it out the first time with your husband, then try it on yourself first. You can try different things and see what you do and do not like. *(Trying some anal stimulation while in the bath tub if you like!)* Then when you talk to your spouse about it, you will already have an idea of what you want and like.

You may even get brave and decide that you'd like to try rimming sometime, which is you licking and kissing the anus.

(Don't look so shocked!) Although some people may find it gross, others will tell you "Don't knock it 'till you've tried it!" I am well aware that some people are not into erotic anal play. You and your spouse will need to talk about it and decide if this is something you are both comfortable trying together. After almost twenty-four years of marriage my wife and I tried it for the first time, and it was amazing. My wife and I weren't virgins when we got married so it was virgin for us, and we both liked it very much. It is now a regular part of our sex life, even when we don't commit to full blown anal sex, we still use fingers, tongues, and toys.

Weighing Your Options

Many naïve Christian couples have no clue that heterosexual couples enjoy anal sex with one another. Many people feel that God did not intend for the anus to be used for penetration of the penis. Its tissue is so vastly different than that of the vagina. It is thinner and tears so easily. Because it is so thin in comparison the thick wall of the vagina. Sperm can easily penetrate the lining which causes the immune system to shut down temporarily. The caution that is needed in order to really minimize the risk of tearing the anal wall and damaging the intended function of the rectum is too much for some warry couples to consider participating in anal sex. Additionally, many others fear the pain of the initial penetration, so they are afraid to try it.

On the other side of the coin there are couples who like to incorporate anal sex into their sex life for a variety of different reasons. All of them valid for their circumstances. For some women who may have given away more of their virtues away to other men prior to marriage and becoming a Christian, it is one thing that they can actually share with their husbands only. Others like my wife love the full feeling of having something in their anus and vagina at the same time. As I said my wife loves this full feeling. This is what is called double penetration. Some find anal stimulation to release their erotic feelings like nothing else. Others want to actually experience something to know if they like it or not. And still others do it just because their spouse likes it, as a gift to them.

I want to really free you up to make your decision of whether or not to participate in anal sex with your spouse based on what you as a couple feel is acceptable for you. The bible is not explicit that anal sex is right or wrong so choose whether or not you will incorporate it based on what God has spoken to your heart about it. And if you do not have clarity, wait. If you disagree with your spouse, talk with them about it without pressure or anger.

The rule of thumb that my wife and I follow is that whoever doesn't wish to incorporate whichever sex act is in question has the deciding vote.   And for all the years in our marriage for whatever reason she said no. Which believe me really surprised me since we are so adventurous in our lovemaking. That is what keeps our sex life so erotic and hot. Each time we make love it is an adventure. However, we continued to talk it through as best we can and try to incorporate things that are uncomfortable for one of us if the other would like to experience it. Having said that, no one should feel pressured to do something that they feel is wrong. That is the key. Find out what God says to YOU about anal sex based on who you and your spouse are as people and make your final decision with that in mind.

You might also be wondering what the appeal is. Sometimes anal sex is really attractive for some because it is forbidden or has an air of naughtiness about it. The anus is a real taboo area for many of us! Other people think than anal sex is great because it offers an extreme tightness, especially for the man. An extremely different set of sensations than vaginal sex. Oh yes it has the amazing promise of highly enjoyable physical sensations.

There are as many reasons for trying anal sex as there are people trying it...but we can make some generalizations.

Anal Play Christians Can Like It Too

Many women like my wife like a bit of anal stimulation during oral sex or masturbation. *(And so, do men, for that matter!) (You can see how it adds to sexual pleasure if you stimulate your own anus with a well-lubed finger when you masturbate.)*

As a man, you should try giving cunnilingus to your wife while you place a finger in her vagina and at the same time gently rub the tip of your little finger on her anus. If she likes this, she'll let you know by her cries of delight as she cums! Basically, the anus and the surrounding area have lots of nerves that link to the clitoris, pelvis, and vulva, so the whole area is extremely sensitive to sexual stimulation and is very sexually responsive. And it CAN feel good if you are penetrated anally. For women, this is an extension of vaginal penetration; for men, there is the excitement that can really be obtained when the prostate gland is stimulated through the wall of the rectum. For men who find that a tight fit produces greater pleasure during sex, the appeal of their partner's anus is quite obvious. But in short - if it excites you, try it out and see if you enjoy it!

Women can also enjoy being taken up the anus, though it's really important that all our experiments are consensual. That is if your partner agrees to whatever you want to do, and you're both happy to draw a boundary line when things get to the point where you want to stop. *(At first my wife would tell me she can't take it today and we would stop and move on to something else just as pleasurable. She has sometimes outbursts from* hemorrhoids from having the kids and sometimes the hemorrhoids say no!)

Always remember, it is clearly not as easy to get your penis into the anus as it is to get it into the vagina, so please do not give up. It will take some practice. Without dodging the issue, if you are worried about poop - and, yes, it can happen that the rectum beyond the anal canal may have some small residue of poop in there when you enter. Then you can do something about it.

First, use a good strong condom. That's pretty much probably a good idea anyway to stop you from getting a urinary tract infection *(bacteria from feces don't mix well with your urethra and kidneys).*

Second, get your partner to take an enema for you before sex. Small douche bags are available from all online sex stores.

Third, have a shower together before you have sex, and wash each other's anuses. That way you get an element of erotic play and relax a bit even before you start. Not long ago my wife and I showered together in a motel and washed each other really good before I gave her analingus and finger play for about an hour, and she exploded several times during the session wanting more.

Chapter 3

Overview of Anal Sex

The greatness of erotic anal sex lies in the fact that stimulating the anus greatly enhances the body's erotic perception. Most people that have tried anal sex are actually surprised by the extremely strong sexual sensation it provides for them. A good lover can make his woman climax from anal sex by stimulating her genitals and clitorus with one hand, and filling her up with the other, she will have that full feeling that will be something special for her.

Anal Sex From a Female Perspective

Anal sex is one of the most erotic and satisfying sexual practices a woman and her husband can enjoy. Anal sex is a different, tighter sensation for the man than vaginal sex. The rectum, once it's ready, literally swallows the penis up and sucks it in and can't get enough of it, believe it or not. If the clitoris and/or vagina are stimulated while your man is inside you, it can take you to another sexual realm in lovemaking. It's pretty intense, no matter what, and the increased tightness back there makes it just that much better.

Oral sex or even intercourse for that matter helps some women to relax and feel at ease before engaging in anal sex. Something that really helps her to relax the anal sphincters is for her man to start rubbing her butt cheeks softly, spreading them gently, and then squeezing them together. Him also teasing her tender anus very slowly with his fingers and tongue makes sure she is very ready.

First you should go very slowly while inserting your penis into her. This allows the anal sphincters to gradually adjust. Secondly, she will really love the erotic sensation of gradually being filled by your penis. It does feel like she's actually swallowing him. Most women like to control the pace by being on top so she is the one to slowly push back on you at the pace they are ready to take you. Anal penetration is an entirely different feeling than vaginal penetration.

There's a lot more pressure for both of you just before actual penetration takes place. It starts with an intense feeling of pressure as the head of his penis presses against her anus, which builds up a feeling of anticipation. Then there is a release of pure pleasure as the head slips through that tight little hole past the sphincters. You really notice the change in diameter as the head moves inside. You feel the length of his slick shaft sliding in with every nerve ending you can imagine. If you're relaxed enough, it feels amazing for the both of you when he gets through the second sphincter.

One of the most exquisite sensations for some women in anal sex is when he pulls out and then slides back in the tight hole for the first time. The in-stroke is intensely sensual. My wife loves slowly at first, but there comes a point where she will want you to speed up and just take her hard and fast. It is then that they feel completely full of your cock. The extremely full sensation is very different from having you in her vagina. Everything is so very tight, and the pressure is what causes the pleasure. The anal passage is being stimulated while at the same time there is pressure on her G-spot through the wall of the vagina. My wife can orgasm rather quickly after penetration, *(whether it be anal beads, butt plugs, a finger, or my penis.)* especially since I usually rub her clitoris once I'm inside her ass. She says it's an amazing feeling to squeeze my penis as her anal muscles tightly contract around me. I usually climax hard as she squeezes me so tightly that I have a hard time moving because the sensation is so intense for us. I've read where some women say when their man ejaculates, it's so much better for them because they can actually feel him shoot his load, whereas, vaginally, they usually can't.

Anal lovemaking can feel absolutely incredible. It's a whole different type of sensation – it's deep inside, it's not the clitoris, and it isn't in the vagina, but feels strangely like both of them in a sort of mixed-up combination in another part of the body. It doesn't feel like anything else you may have felt before. Women who don't enjoy anal sex are probably doing it wrong.

One of the worst things that can happen to any man is not being "sure" if he has finally given his woman a climax. Over 70% of women claim that their partners have never given them an actual orgasm with intercourse, and even 65% of women admit to faking orgasms. Just imagine being so sexually skilled that you can literally have any woman screaming with pleasure and sexually exhausted from a night of giving her orgasm after orgasm.

Chapter 4

Preparation for The Exploration

Your rectum can actually receive a large penis easily and fully. After all think about it folks it stretches wide to accommodate your large turds. And beside instead of taking a dump a penis can be quite pleasurable, if you want it. And you must want it, before it can actually happen. That is, you must be at ease, in mind and body. The rectum is similar to a very elastic pipe with a set of muscular rings at the end of the anus. The anus acts as a plug, to stop things from going out, or letting them in. It tightens and relaxes like purse strings on a bag and is fairly strong as well.

This muscle is actually controlled by the mind. Did you see that? Let me say it again. It's really important that you do not miss this point of you want your anal sex experience to be fun and pleasurable for you as well. This muscle is controlled by the mind, and our emotions influence how tense it will be at any given time. Good non painful anal penetration can't happen unless the anus is totally relaxed, and this may take some learning on her part. Many of us are taught to be ashamed of our rear ends, because of the things that happen there.

The anus can also be a truly erotic place. Most children experience pleasure in going to the bathroom, but many adults ignore these feelings, in their rush to get the act over with and feel as little guilt as possible. The rear end then becomes an ignored and very mysterious place. The anus is usually held tight and becomes the site of problems like hemorrhoids. Yet the feelings are still there. But no matter what awareness and conscious control of the anus can be learned, although this takes time to discover. Look at it as exploring some new, part of your own body.

Exploring Your Own Private Butthole

The first thing you must decide for yourself is how do you personally feel about your own anus and rectum? Are they a part of you, or do you emotionally push them away? If you feel bad about your rosebud, *(my pet name for my wife's butthole)* you feel that it's a dirty place, then this is where your explorations must begin. Explore your own anus when you are alone, to discover how it feels and that it's not dirty. You can touch it and you will see that it does not hurt, so you must not feel embarrassed. You can do this in two ways: by yourself or with your lover. In exploring by yourself you have complete control over your actions. Climb into a tub of hot water *(or a shower and when you are clean lay on your bed)* and relax. Then with your fingertips explore your vulva and thighs, gliding around them to feel what it's like. Then bend your legs and tenderly slide your fingers down between them, sliding them along the crack that runs from your vulva to your anus. Touch your anus very lightly with one finger. Then try with several fingers pushing down a little - how does it feel? If you like that then try masturbating while pressing several fingers on the outside of your butthole.

Finally, after you've made direct contact with it. If it feels good there or if you sense that it will, keep feeling good; Okay ... Don't push yourself to do more than you want at this point.

Making First Contact

Now that you've made contact. If it feels good touching it or if you sense that it will, keep exploring. Don't push yourself to do more than you want at any one time - pace yourself comfortably. But try to tune in on your butthole; discover when it's tight and when it's loose, and how you can control this. At some point you'll want to take the plunge, inserting a finger inside. It's a remarkable discovery, that you can do this, and believe me my friends it opens up a world of new sensations. You'll discover that the rectum is a sturdy, flexible organ and can't be hurt by fingers, or a penis or other similar objects, unless you violently intend to do so. Sharp edges like fingernails can scratch it, and that's not good, so guys trim your nails a little first. *(for ladies with long fingernails take a latex glove and place a cotton ball under your fingernail and place the glove on over it and lube it up and you're ready for penetration.)*

Remember ladies your ass is big enough, if it can take all your excrement, it can take on smaller things like fingers and penises. Usually there's nothing inside the very end-part of the rectum. But sometimes there might be some small particles. You'll discover that these are quite harmless and easily washed off after you are finished. Or you can clean out your rectum first, by douching it with an enema bottle and warm water.

Now, I suggest you to lie back on your bed (or wherever) and bend your legs to bring your feet up close to your rear. Get into an enjoyable masturbation session with one hand and grease a finger of the other with KY or another lubricant. Then place it at your anus and push very gently, and slowly. Your finger will go in just a little. If you want to get your finger in farther, you must keep pushing gently and firmly, and release the anal muscle.

Then you will actually feel your finger go all the way through, past the thick muscle and into the soft, juicy tender rectum. It may feel uncomfortable at first, because you've taught yourself to regard anything in the rectum as dark and dirty, and you'll want to push it out. But take it easy; try letting your finger rest there as you're masturbating. You may feel a little burning or irritation at first, but this will turn into pleasure if your masturbation is feeling good. If you like, go ahead and come to a climax with your finger inside, and see how it feels. If all this seems good to you, keep up the exploration. If it bothers you, withdraw and try again later when you're feeling more adventurous, just take your time.

Loosening Up

Now you'll want to learn to loosen your anus enough to let in larger sized objects. It may seem at first like your anus has a separate personality, doing things in its own way. But this is only because you have separated it in your mind. If you get to know it better, it'll eventually make good friends with you, and the separation will disappear. After using your finger to meet it, get to know your anus more intimately and more often. In fact the more you touch it and play with it the more it becomes stretched and ready for bigger and better activities.

You can also trace warm wet rings around the outside of the anus. After inserting a finger, you can massage it, pressing outward in a circle, tensing, and calming it, trying to curl your finger around its side, feeling its touch through the skin. While exploring, if you act like you are pooping, or pushing out, this will help you get used to the feeling even more. Practice stretching and tensing/calming your anus around your finger. You may want to do this until it can be widened easily and painlessly. Next you can insert two (or more) fingers, seeing how far you can bend them apart.

Later, on you might want to try a dildo *(a straight, smooth, round tipped object like those found in sex shops)*. It's a good idea to use something that won't break, such as plastic or rubber. My wife and I prefer butt plugs of various sizes to stretch her ass with. Otherwise feel free to indulge, since you can only hurt your rectum by using sharp objects or violent jabbing motions.

More Experimenting With Your Partner

From the very beginning you might want to move right on to experimenting with your spouse. And this is also another way to learn about your own butthole. Say to him "I'd sure like to enjoy some anal pleasures tonight, but I'm not used to it and a little afraid," Then your husband can turn you on. He can place his fingers at your anus during regular or oral sex. He can if he likes, suck and tongue your anus, or insert his finger(s). These actions are called analingus and postillioning, and can be soothing, warm, and exciting.

Another nice thing for your husband to do is to masturbate you as his finger is inserted in your rectum. *(My wife's favorite thing)* If neither of you can get this far because your anus just won't relax, it means you're anxious or you simply don't know how to relax it yet. This is not always the easiest thing to learn, and there's no reason to feel bad about it, since the anus is very likely to just follow old habits of not opening up. It takes time. Take risks only when you really feel safe, and don't allow yourself to be forced open. It helps to talk about this, and how you're feeling.

One especially nice act that can relax your rear is for your husband, during sex, to simply trace soft rings around the opening, pressing with one or two lubricated fingertips, going around and around. This usually has a calming effect. If, after much gentle trying over a period of time, your anus just won't loosen, I would suggest you might have a mental wish not to be entered that you aren't aware of. If this might be the case, explore the possibility in your mind and with your partner. You may want to just forget about anal sex altogether and move on to all the other great sex acts God gave us to enjoy like oral sex and using different positions in vaginal sex. But if you do actually progress in your explorations, the time will come for your husband to insert his penis. If this is what you both want, let it happen, as it will, without planning on doing it. *(Every time my wife and I plan it, it doesn't work out, but sometimes she just wants it and she'll lube up my penis and we'll just go at it.)* Be easy about it, trying one of the positions we'll discuss later on in this book.

It may take several (or many) tries, so relax and feel the sensations. *(It took many tries for me and my wife and lots of fun laughing as I got soft trying to get it in. That little bugger is really tight sometimes.)* If it hurts, and it might, just ask him to withdraw gently, but not completely. Some pain may happen, and this is usually okay. If it's a strong or sharp pain, back off. You will discover that the mild pain turns to blissful delight during sex. As he enters, you may experience a sudden urge to go to the bathroom, or you may imagine you're going to urinate or poop right there.

This is a fantasy of your mind and body, through lack of use and conditioning; if you respect these feelings and have patience, they will change through practice. Also, if you're sexually excited these feelings and any tightness will lessen considerably. The best rule is to take it in steps, going easy and smooth. It may seem difficult for a while , but you may be surprised by a rapid change from discomfort to sweet pleasure.

Chapter 5

Anal Pleasure's Long History

Millions of people even Christians practice and enjoy anal play every day.

Anal sex has a rich history of being practiced by many people, as it is a well-known fact, that people of many ancient cultures preferred anal sex to a vaginal intercourse. Many only practicing vaginal intercourse just to procreate. However, the attitude towards anal intercourse and anal eroticism always depended on the culture and religion of a particular nation.

While it was widely spread and highly praised by ancient people, the introduction of puritan Christianity to the United States affected the attitude towards anal sex a lot. The incorrect attitudes of the early puritan's created the negative attitude and made a huge impact on the United States, affecting Europe to a lesser degree. Even nowadays the attitude toward anal sex of the majority of people in America is very negative. The society still considers it to be unnatural, indecent, and improper behavior.

Despite the society's negative attitude, there is nothing politically incorrect about anal sex. It is simply just one of the many variants of sexual intercourse that couples can share together. Another main fallacy about anal sex is that only homosexuals can enjoy it. However, many healthy heterosexual couples are now practicing anal play too and enjoying it as well. The major concerns people have about anal intercourse are safety and the painful sensation. To dispel these worries we can say that anal sex is safe and won't cause be a very painful experience if performed in a correct way. The length and width of human rectum exceed the average size of a man's penis and anal sex won't turn into a painful experience if you don't apply too much force. If you made up your mind to try this type of play, it would be better if your partner has a long penis but with a small girth size. That will ease the insertion into your rectum. But if you still have concerns that your husband's penis is too big for your anus, you can always use anal toys instead. And slowly work your way up to his size penis or not. This is the best solution for first time anal intercourse, as you can also choose the size to use and can control the frequency, force, and depth of penetration.

Another advantage to using anal toys is that you can use them during the vaginal intercourse with your partner or during clitoral stimulation or even both for that matter. You can also let your partner penetrate you anally with a dildo or an anal vibrator, which is also a very pleasurable experience for both of you. In fact, my wife loves to penetrate me anally with a dildo while she is giving me fellatio. And finally, using anal toys gives you (the wife) an opportunity to introduce anal play to your man and let him experience some anal pleasure of his own.

There are few things that you have to remember about anal sex. Always use special lubrication when inserting something in your rectum, whether it be a penis or anal toy. Don't try to fully insert a penis or a dildo during your first-time of doing anal play. Start introducing some minor anal play into your sex life slowly, by experimenting with small anal toys and butt plugs to find out what works best for you. We started with a graduated butt plug kit and worked out way up from there. You will know when it is time to move on up to a penis.

Chapter 6

How Should You Approach Your Partner's Anal Opening?

For men getting started …Simply start with a finger.

A nice way to start is to play with a fingertip on or around your wife's anus. You can then rub gently, pressing into the rosebud *(my pet name for my wife's butthole)* opening. Tickle it gently with your fingertip, and then with enough anal lube gently start the act of penetration to get her relaxed and opened up a bit. Such play is good for both sexes, so hopefully you'll let her do the same thing to you. This will increase her confidence and may make the whole thing am lot more fun. It then becomes a game of equality rather than something you are just doing to her. That knowledge may give her greater pleasure when you finally get to enter her with your penis.

The other thing we should bear in mind is that many people find some sexual acts acceptable only when they are highly aroused. So, if you both get really turned on and start getting carried away with the idea of anal sex, don't forget all the rules about going slow, being well lubricated and maybe even using a condom!

To sum it up: start the act of anal play with a gentle fingertip, tickling and pressing until your lover begins to open up and relax a little. You might even consider using your tongue on her anus, though this is definitely something that either appeals to you or doesn't. Provided you're both completely well and healthy, it should be okay health wise, but there may be a slight risk of hepatitis or other nasty infections, so take your choice and risk as you will. You may find it's appealing to use your tongue, you may not. But without prejudging the issue, what's certainly true from my own personal experience is that it can be highly erotic and exciting for some people to have a warm wet tongue probing this most intimate area of their body.

Other Issues To Deal With Anal Sex

Unless you're playing out some real masochistic game, pain should not be part of the agenda. And anal sex can be really painful without enough lube for the person on the receiving end! Never in any sex act is there more consideration required for your partner than in anal sex. If she is in discomfort at any time, use more lube or just stop. And that's especially true if she's so nervous that she just can't open up enough for you to get in. Time and patience and a gentle finger - or two - may be the answer or they may not. But if you can't penetrate her easily, don't force the issue - either psychologically or physically!

It's so very important for us to remember that sometimes during anal intercourse, the receiving partner may have a reflex response which feels like they need to go and take a dump. If this happens to you, you may find that stopping for a moment or two makes the urge go away - or, if god forbid it does develop into a full-blown need to go to the bathroom, then that's probably the end of your anal play for the night!

More for Men

There are two very tight rings of muscle around the anal canal, one at the outside, and one on the inside. The first one will open up quite easily for you, but the second one may clamp shut if your partner is a little frightened or apprehensive, or you go too fast. That's its job - to prevent things from getting into the body from the outside. The way to overcome this is to press forward slowly with plenty of lube *(don't forget, you've already gone in with a finger or two, so it knows what's coming - and so does your partner!)*. At some point, if your lover is basically accepting of the idea of being penetrated anally, the inner muscles will relax and allow your penis to enter her body easily. If they don't, make sure you're not causing her any pain, and stop if she wants you to do so.

By the way friend, the best way to get in is to get down there and watch what you are doing. It's not like the vagina, where you may be able to just put your penis in the general area and penetrate her without even looking. Her anus doesn't have labia lips to guide your penis in, and the opening is not as big as that of the vulva channel into the vagina. Simply you will need to look at it to be able to penetrate it! And you need to apply a steady pressure as you seek to get your penis into her.

Gentle but very firm is the watchword here. You can push forward, and then pull backwards a bit, and then the next time, go a bit further forward. Obviously, such a movement will be easier in some positions than others. Like the rear entry with her kneeling on the bed in front of you and you standing behind her, for example. Once she is experienced and confident and can relax to allow you in her at will. Believe me it will get easier with practice and confidence.

How Hard Can You Thrust At First?

Well, the simple answer is as hard as your wife lets you! Move slowly and lovingly, thrusting gently until she is used to it and accepting of the rhythm of your penile thrusting. You may also find it enough to move slowly and gently with restricted thrusts, or you may want to go at it full pelt. In either case, make sure your wife is both willing and able to accept your thrusts. Never forget it is a special and delicate part of her body, and she deserves your care and respect *(not to mention your thanks)* for giving you the amazing opportunity to enjoy such a tight fit of her body around your penis. We know it feels good to have a tight penetration - we're men. Remember it may not feel as good for her as it does for you!

For the Women

If you can relax and enjoy the thrusting, fine. But if it hurts and you want your partner to withdraw, tell him to stop immediately! There's no reason why you should have to accept this form of sex if you don't like it. But remember there is always a little bit of pain or I should say a light burning at the initial contact, but it does go away and give way to some pretty incredible pleasure if you can take the initial burn.

Other Points To Consider

You may also find a little bit of blood. That is some small rips and cuts are common consequences of anal intercourse. Stop participating in this act until they heal, and next time use a lot more lube, and relax more as you play with all the different the positions that are available to you. If the condom you are using breaks, simply stop and get a new one, put it on, lube all up and start again. If you're going on to orgasm, and ejaculate your cum inside your lover, make sure the condom is intact before you cum, or else she may have a runny stool for several days.

It is just possible that after a while you might want to completely shift positions entirely and have a session of anal sex where the woman penetrates the man. That way she can get some sense of what it's like to be the dominant partner who penetrates during sex.

Second, he gets his prostate massaged by his wife's lubed up finger or the dildo or butt plug, and if she simultaneously masturbates him, he may find that he cums in a tremendous orgasm. I have like most men had my most powerful orgasms when my wife does this. Certainly, massaging his prostate *(easiest in the rear entry position where the man kneels with his butt in the air, opening his cheeks so she can penetrate him from behind)* this will also increase the volume of his semen that he produces, and make his ejaculation shoot a lot further and harder, and give him greater orgasmic pleasure. It's certainly going to be a new experience for him! And believe me my wife has used a butt plug and her fingers on me while she gives me fellatio and it makes me explode longer and more intense.

Most women will also like stimulation of the anus toward the area of her tender G-spot. The truth is that membrane between the anus and the vagina is very thin. Combining anal and G-Spot Stimulation adds to the sensual feeling for women.

Because the G-spot is analogous to the prostate gland in men. He will like this upper area also touched as well. Feel for the prostate gland. Hold pressure here when stimulating the man.

Chapter 7

Anal Play vs Anal Sex?

Usually when people think of anal sex they think of penis penetration. This is but one part of anal play. In fact, my wife and I rarely partake in penis penetration, but we always have some form of anal play. Anal play is so erotic! Now if you're not interested in penis penetration, it doesn't mean you have to ignore this entire part of your body. This whole area of the body has been largely ignored for its sexual potential. The bum, the anus, and the rectum are all sites of enormous potential pleasure for us.

In fact, these areas of the body are the second most powerful erogenous zone for a woman only taking a backseat to her clitoris. And they respond to feelings of touch, pressure, movement, and can be incredibly pleasurable. As you read on in the future chapters most of the time we're going to be talking about anal penis penetration; but there's a lot that we can explore about the anus without actually going inside it.

Working From The Outside Inward

Start by carefully exploring your partner's entire backside with your hands and fingers. Massage their bum cheeks and once you've got your gloves and lube on you can start gently touching and massaging the anal opening.

Don't rush to penetration, and don't stampede to the anus like a herd of horses. Instead pay attention to how their body is responding to all the different kinds of touches you are using. Try a slow circular massaging motion with your fingers or gently knead the skin and muscle underneath. Take note of where they like to be touched, and where they can handle a more vigorous stimulation versus a softer touch.

Pushing Not Poking

Listen to this important fact. Never force a penis or dildo into the anus. Using what you learned during your mutual anal exploration sessions press the tip gently against the anal opening and wait for your wife to relax and let you in. Keep stimulating your wife at the same time with your hands or with a sex toy. When you're having anal sex with your wife, providing clitoral stimulation is a good idea.

Also pay close attention to how your partner is moving and move with them, not against, them. The amazing thing about the human body is that once your wife's sphincter muscles finally relax, you'll suddenly feel yourself being drawn inside her. It will actually suck your penis inside her smoothly and softly. *(And yes, this feels really amazing because it is so tight)* Remember to only let yourself slide in as much as your wife's body allows you to.

Just Be There For Her

Once you have penetrated your wife's bum the first time, do not immediately begin thrusting in and out or even moving very much at all for that matter. Just take a moment to feel what it's like and to let your honey get comfortable with the full feeling and some penetration. After a few minutes the burning sensation will end.

Don't forget to keep all the other kinds of stimulation that you are doing going *(I'm talking about, using your hands on her breasts or clitoris, and using sex toys fellas).* If your wife is moving her body, you can then gently move with her. Unless she knows how deep she wants it, don't try to penetrate her deeper until you're both really turned on even more.

How to Move… Once you're both completely comfortable then slowly begin to experiment with some different types of movements. Start moving slowly inside of her trying both in/out and maybe some side-to-side movements. Pay close attention to how her body is responding to your movements *(also, you can ask her). After a while when you find something that works for both of you, then you can begin to ramp up the intensity slowly.* Anal penetration is not like vaginal penetration, and it has to build up slower and may never be as vigorous. If your wife is unsure, you can then ask her to do the moving at first and you keep your body still. You can also suggest she be on top if she would like to control the thrusting. Although in this position it will be hard for her to relax the anus.

Postillioning

There are a couple of ways to get your partner involved in the exploration of your butthole. They are called pistoling and analingus.

Pistoling is simply the insertion of fingers into the anus and may also involve tenderly massaging it and the rectum. The insertion of your partner's fingers into your anus is a great lead up to the ultimate of anal sex or it can even be a really pleasant enhancement to us having regular intercourse. This also allows your wife to become familiar with how you may react during anal sex. It gives him a chance to explore your body with you. Normally, I find that the index or middle fingers work the best, being a little longer than the others of them and stronger as well. Don't forget the lube! Run your fingers all over the anal opening, kneading, and pressing against it. You can use a circular motion if you would like. It's just like giving a massage. You are helping the area around the anus to relax. Make the insertion by very carefully pressing gently and firmly inwards. Then you can wiggle the tip of your finger as necessary.

At this point if your partner is comfortable and relaxed the finger should slide in fairly easily. On the other hand, if the butthole is tense then your finger will not make any headway at all. You and your wife will have to decide at this point whether or not to continue or to perhaps leave it alone and come back to it another time.

Once your finger is past the anal opening you will feel the thick, strong, muscular ring which is the anus and beyond it, the soft sides of the rectum. You will need to keep at least your fingertip beyond the anus, or the contraction of the muscle could just force the finger right out. When your finger is finally inside exploring a bit, pushing the finger as far in as it will go, flicking back and forth. Just go slow at first. A great way to enhance this exploration would be to suck on your wife's clit or stick your other fingers in her vagina. I have found that this combination makes for some pretty powerful orgasms. There is nothing better than having my mouth wrapped around her clit and my fingers wiggling in her rosebud. It's a great feeling my wife tells me. (*as if I can't tell by her moaning*)

Check In With Her Often

Be sure to check in with your wife often during anal sex. You can do this easily verbally by asking *(is that good? Do you like that? Do you want more, less, different? etc....)* and you can ask your honey to give you feedback without you asking *(more, slow it down, let's try this, harder, etc....)* You can also get a lot of information from what's happening non-verbally with their body's reactions. Are they tensing up? Are they moving around more? Is her breathing becoming heavier, deeper, and shallower? Is she getting wetter? All of this information can also help you get into a rhythm with her and speed up, slow down, or keep going.

Chapter 8

Maybe It's Time For More Than Fingers

Now that you are comfortable with fingers, it's time to move on to something a bit more realistic. A good dildo is excellent to practice with. You can obtain one at a love shop or order from many places on the internet. *(Covenant spice is a good non-pornographic Christian website for those looking for one.)* I would recommend one made of plastic rather than latex. Latex dildos are difficult to clean and have soft pores that bacteria could be harbored in. Don't use anything with sharp edges or that can easily break.

If you do use latex, it's best to cover it with a condom before you use it. On your own try inserting the dildo into your butt gradually, making sure that it is well lubricated. Try pushing it in and out of your anus while you masturbate yourself with the other hand. I have found that if my wife is already excited from me masturbating her with my fingers it is much simpler to push the butt plug or dildo further into her anus.

Overcoming Normal Fears

One of the biggest problems for an anal virgin is the terrible fear that the man's penis will be too big to penetrate comfortably. The reality is that with us using lots of good quality lube, and using just a slow steady pressure, penetration can be quite easy. But you do need to be in a certain *state of mind* before it will happen with ease. It's all about her relaxing, and opening up, and her knowing that her body can take it, and being willing to accept penetration in this way. Once you've got over that hurdle, anal penetration can be easy, as the body tends to respond with relaxation of the anal sphincter when required.

The truth is it's actually quite normal for the muscles of the anus to clamp tight when it is being pushed at from the outside. But provided the muscles are being properly relaxed even the biggest penis will fit in easily. The key to painless anal sex is to relax your muscles naturally, completely, and the best way to learn to do this is to practice it on your own. *(Of course, if you're particularly uninhibited, there's absolutely no reason why you shouldn't play round together with your partner, but that does require a measure of openness and intimacy which you may not feel comfortable with. But let me tell you friends if you want to have a wonderful sex life you must make it an open experience for the two of you.*

My wife and I are open to pleasing the other and aside from beating the other with some kind of whip (not a small paddle) or adding other people to the mix, there isn't a whole lot we won't try at least once.)

If you find that you need to persevere to learn how to relax your anal sphincters, and you still want to try anal penetration, my advice to you would be not to give up too soon. Anal intercourse can also be very rewarding and bring a special level of pleasure to sex, but the reason most people give it up is because they haven't truly learned the art of relaxing their anal sphincters. Admittedly, even when you're experienced in the art of anal penetration it is still possible to feel a small amount of pain at the moment of penetration. The difference is that you don't clamp down tight in fear when you're an experienced anal penetrator. Instead, you try to relax even more, as your partner stops pushing, and you wait until the pain or burning subsides. After which you can then resume the penetration more enjoyably. So, you might also want to practice initially with a dildo or better yet a butt plug. Perhaps even get a series of dildos or butt plugs of increasing size, until you're comfortable with the anal penetration. Follow these simple steps and you will have a great experience with your lover.

Step one: Cleaning It All Up

Women that are on the receiving end are very likely to be worried about their cleanliness. Not just because it's aesthetically distasteful to have a penis covered with dodo, but also because on a more practical level poop can be quite abrasive to her and lead to a soreness if penetration is without sufficient lube. If you happen to know that you passed all the material in your colon when you go to the toilet, you may need to do nothing more than simply wash the area thoroughly on the outside of your anus. If you're in any doubt at all about how clean you are internally, you can then put a well lubed finger up through your anal sphincters and just feel around whether or not there are small particles of waste matter left inside.

But if you want to be 100% certain that you've got them all cleaned out it's very easy enough to get a suitable anal douche from an online sex shop. It's advisable not to use an enema right before you do it because the quantity of water you put in is so great that you may find some of it gets trapped, only to emerge at a very inconvenient moment when you're enjoying intercourse. In any event, it's a very good idea to have a thick towel underneath you so that you can catch anything, whether it be liquid or solid that might happen to emerge as you enjoy sex.

Step two: Turning Her On With Foreplay

The whole idea of foreplay is simply to turn you on so that you are both relaxed in body and mind and accept the idea of anal penetration. *(Many people find ideas that are not acceptable when they are not aroused become very attractive when they're sexually aroused, and nowhere is this truer than in anal play.)* The very idea of which may be a turnoff in the initial stages of sex but seem very appealing after you are aroused. If you're an experienced butthole penetrator you may even find that during foreplay you feel your anal sphincters relaxing in anticipation of penetration, as well as experiencing the mental or emotional desire to be penetrated.

Step three: Rimming Around The Anus

Rimming as we have already said is the word used for licking around your lover's butt hole, and even penetrating it with the tip of your tongue. If you're a woman learning to be penetrated, you can get an idea of what it might feel like by using gentle fingertip pressure on your anal sphincter while you masturbate. Perhaps later on even building up to full finger penetration in a rhythmic way, as though you were being screwed.

If you are a willing man, it's well worth exploring the sensations you get by adding a little bit of anal play with a finger to your masturbatory experience: If you do try this you will probably find it enhances your sensations considerably.

When you're sexually aroused, it's a great idea to lick around the rim of your partner's butthole, using plenty of saliva as lubrication. At some point you may feel you want to explore by penetrating gently with the tip of your tongue, an act which is likely to make your partner want further penetration.

Please we must also bear in mind that this kind of intimate play may increase your chances of you getting an infection such as hepatitis from your lover who may be a hepatitis carrier without knowing it. So, if anal play will be a big part of your sex life -- and arguably if it's any part of your sex life -- then you might consider getting inoculated to protect yourself against hepatitis.

Step four: Lubing Your Finger and Penetrating Your Lover's Anus

Using your fingers to open her up a little before you penetrate her with our penis. This is a gentle way of making sure that your partner is relaxed. Since you can start with one finger and move up to as many as three, it's a good way of ensuring that she's open and ready for penetration with your penis. If you use a dildo instead of fingers, remember to cover it first with a condom, and don't share it together to avoid the transmission of infection. If you practice with a dildo, make sure you've got one that is less than 5 inches round, which is about 1.5 inches across in diameter, and certainly much less than 7 inches long. If you use anything much bigger than this, it is not going to help you learn how to relax easily.

My wife and I prefer different size butt plugs that gradually get bigger. When we first started with my wife the smallest one was just right and after a little while it kept falling out when she got really aroused so we went on to the next size, and so on. Now she really enjoys a real long 8inch butt vibrator. She goes crazy with it inside her rear. *(And please, do everything you can to avoid an embarrassing trip to the emergency room to extract a can of deodorant, or some other foreign object that you've decided to use for a spot of anal stimulation: while the hospital staff will have seen it all before, you can spare yourself considerable embarrassment if you stick to sex toys and use them sensibly. In this context, it's a good idea if you use a butt plug with a wide base so that it can't penetrate further than it's meant to.)*

Step five: Penetration With Penis In A Condom

When you are both ready, have the penetrating husband roll a condom down over his erection and add ample lubrication. Remember this motto: too much lubrication is just enough. If you want a try sex without a condom *(so-called bareback sex)* like me then you really have to be 110% sure of your lover's HIV status. Anal sex is the easiest way to transmit the HIV infection, and infection rates are now increasing again as people becomes more blasé about the risks of unprotected sex.

So how do you start your journey into anal penetration without anxiety or stress?

When you have finally achieved full penetration, you can move into other positions, but the element of control that is implicit in this erotic position may lessen anxiety from the partner who is receiving. You might also find that doggie style, where the wife kneels on all fours is more comfortable for both her and you. And another favorite for many is simply the classic missionary position, with her legs lifted up high to your sides.

In all of these amazing positions, the wife, lets her husband gently press the tip of his erection against her butthole. Add plenty of lube, and each time that he presses the tip of his erection against your butt hole, allow it to open wider and wider. He may also feel your ass muscles are resisting at first, but it's important that at this stage in the action you don't panic, or experience anxiety about what's happening, because with just slow and steady pressure your anus will certainly relax and open up. Also remember that any tightness wrapped around his manhood can induce men to have a faster orgasm, so men beware. *(I remember my first time we had full penetration I was so excited; I just got the head in her butt and blew my load.)*

At the point where your muscles do finally relax and your husband manages to penetrate through your inner sphincter, you may also feel a little bit of pain, burning or discomfort. If this happens, quickly ask your husband to stop and wait until these muscle spasms end. It's nice for the receiving partner to have the penetrating partner push their penis in and out slowly and gently, withdrawing and then pushing a little bit further in each time. Such slow insertion can be very erotic and exciting.

When you've finally achieved a deep and full penetration, it's really important that the husband remains motionless for a while so that her muscles around the anus can relax. At this point you can then start a rhythmical screwing in and out. If you're not comfortable, ask your husband to adjust the speed and angle of his thrusting. You'll very quickly find that you're now experiencing extreme pleasure rather than discomfort. In fact, this is a highly erotic area, and the potential for sexual pleasure is considerable. Both men and women have nerve networks which surround the anal area and connect with nerves from the highly sensitive prostate and penis in men, and the clitoris and vagina in women. Having said that; believe me it's not unusual for a woman to reach orgasm through anal stimulation alone. My wife literally explodes after very little anal stimulation. If she is having a hard time reaching an orgasm all I have to do is insert and finger in her anus and she will soon be blowing her load. Most women and it is quite a few who are open to the whole experience will at least feel pleasure from the stimulation of this sensitive area, but it may need a few tries before the pleasure overcomes the apprehension or the inhibition that we associate with touching the anal area.

For most women there is also a lot of excitement of being penetrated, which can be a powerful erotic stimulus for most woman - and indeed for her lover. Because men simply love penetration, we were made to penetrate. So, we can assume for both sexes the act of penetration, whether it is it vaginal or anal is linked to some fundamental sexual pleasures. By the way, anal sex may not be so good for you if you're a man that struggles with the problem of premature ejaculation. The tightness of the anus, compared to the vagina, means this tendency may be made even worse! The asshole is very tight fellows!

Chapter 9

Understand The Anatomy of The 2 Sphincters

As we have already said there are two tight rings of muscles in the anus, one external, and one deeper. You can feel them if you put your finger inside the anal canal about an inch deep and then press against the side of the canal. They are less than an inch apart.

And while the woman may control the external sphincter, she has very little control over the deeper inside one, which has to relax unconsciously. It is simply a reflex contraction so that even when a woman says she is relaxed and willing, her internal anal sphincter muscle may determine otherwise. You need to be really patient with her and allow your wife's mind and body plenty of time to relax. It may help to try positions to enable it to happen.

Stimulate the anal region while you enter her

For some people touching the anus or rectum alone may feel very uncomfortable for either partner. But when you do it at the same time as you are doing vaginal penetration or oral sex, it will feel much better.

For example, while you are making love to her vaginally, you can also use a dildo or another sex toy in your wife's anus to give her the sensation of double penetration and of course she can insert a sex toy into her man's anus as he penetrates her or as she's doing oral sex on him. It's up to you to decide what you'd like to try.

Anal stimulation has also been proposed as a cure for a man's delayed ejaculation, because it provides a whole bunch more stimulation to him. That's just a suggestion - though there is no real evidence to back this up.

So, assuming you have gone quite slowly, and gently, you will probably now be deep inside your lover's bowels, connected in a very special way. Anal sex is a privilege for a man and I think it demands a lot from a woman, as it can be a real test of trust. Having said that, many women do actually enjoy it and it can also become a regular feature of a couple's sex life. So, once you've both got used to it, and she is able to relax sufficiently, that is to let her anus admit you and accommodate your thrusting, you may be wondering now what is next. I guess you can try other positions that will allow you to kiss, fondle and hold each other while you are inside her. One example of this would be to have the woman get on top while she straddles you.

This is amazing position where the man can thrust gently and intermittently so as to extend the time before he cums. While at the same time he can reach her vagina and massage her G spot and clit with his fingers or thumb. This could also be helpful in allowing a couple to reach simultaneous orgasm - it's certainly worth a try.

Always Obey the Rules of Hygiene

There is a good reason why women have to wipe their bottoms from the front to back – that is poop may cause bad vaginal infections. So, when your penis or fingers have been in or on her anus, you must not put them in the vagina unless you discard the condom you used for anal sex and use a new one for vaginal entry.

Thoroughly wash your fingers and hands before you use them on her sensitive vagina. In short, go from the vagina to the anus, but not from anus to vagina.

By following these careful tips, anal love can be really fun and safe. You personally need to be absolutely comfortable in both your mind and body, so if she is squeamish about something, simply just find out why. Make sure you effectively communicate about your desires and wishes. This always brings you closer as a couple and enhances your sex life.

Do Men Enjoy Anal Penetration?

And by that I actually do not mean, "Do men enjoy penetrating a woman anally?" But instead, I mean, do men enjoy the sensation of being penetrated anally by a finger, a vibrator, or a sex toy? You must cautiously break the stigma that associates anal sex with homosexuality. *(A false connection in any case.)* Think instead of the simple erotic pleasure that a man or woman may feel when an area of the body is so richly endowed with thousands of nerve endings and very closely associated with sexual pleasure. As they receives stimulation from a loving spouse.

And then let us think one step further. A step which carefully takes you inside the man's anus and into his rectum. That place where his highly sensitive prostate gland resides, that lies within reach of his lover's finger. And with that simple fact comes the possibility of a whole range of pleasure which a man may receive from having his prostate gland stimulated in the proper way. Is that anal sex? Certainly! Is it homosexual? Indeed not!

Since we all have a God given right to take sexual pleasure from our bodies, this seems to us to be a legitimate way of getting sexual satisfaction.

We'll Come Back To This Idea Later....

Though, many times already in this book I have given you some essential warnings about anal sex. Clearly, the anus is potentially a route to infection, if dodo happens to come into contact with the urethra or vagina - and the first of those applies equally to men and women. So, if you use a finger, or a sex toy, or a penis, to penetrate an anus, then you must avoid using that same object to later penetrate either your partner's anus or vagina. You can use a small douche, easily available on-line from sex stores, to wash out any small particles of poop which may be residing in the rectum. Or you can just ignore this and accept the fact that you may connect with some excrement and simply wash it off later. Obviously, latex gloves or finger cots are another great alternative. *(Our favorite)*

The chief reason, in my view, to use a douche or enema before anal play is to avoid the rather unpleasant smell that comes from feces when it meets semen. There is also the possibility that penetrating your wife may trigger a reflex reaction that causes them to need to empty their bowel. This is simply a matter of getting accustomed to having something go up the rectum instead of down and out. A great way to get really comfortable with the whole idea of anal lovemaking is to wash in the shower before you play. As you do so, run your finger around the inside of your anus to make sure it's completely clean. After that, be relaxed, and avoid any cross contamination or mouth or vaginal contact, and you'll be fine.

So now, for the sake of our own conscience and completeness, is the standard warning you see about anal sex. Don't put anything in the vagina or the mouth that you have inserted into the anus, so that you can avoid transferring any bacteria or hepatitis viruses.

Anal Sex Needs Lots of Lubrication

Lubrication is not an option; it is very necessary for comfortable anal sex. Whether you are simply playing around inside your lover's body or on the outside, you will need lots of lubrication. When you're on the outside, for example that is when you're tenderly massaging your lover's anus, you can just use saliva as a lube. But as soon as you start to play around with deep penetration, you need a good quality lube such as olive oil or massage oil, or coconut oil, or some type of a commercial sex lube. For example, ID Glide, Probe or Astroglide. Unfortunately, oil, despite its enjoyable slippery properties, will quickly render a latex condom completely useless. Or you can just go bareback (No condom) My favorite- for my wife wants to feel my load explode inside her.

Water-based lubricants such as Astroglide or Probe can be restored to full slipperiness when they dry out by the simple addition of a little water. Always, always, when you are going into the anus, where there is no natural lube, use as much artificial lube as you need to be comfortable. Anal sex should not be painful for either partner or even uncomfortable for that matter. That is if you are both going to enjoy it.

Just add a generous dose of lube and then add some more. And always be ready to use more if your partner expresses any discomfort. Having said that, as you may already know, too much lube reduces friction to the point where there can be no sensation. And in my experience, some lubes actually numb sensation anyway, so you may need to experiment to find the ideal solution for you and your partner.

Cleaning Her Up Afterwards

Even if you can't see it, there may be some residue fecal matter and bacteria that can and will be spread to other parts of your body if you touch them after touching the outside or inside of her anus. Remember as I've already stated you should never move from anal play to vaginal play without washing carefully first. A bacterium that lives happily in the anus is not happy in the vagina and can cause serious infection. Below are some tips on cleaning up after anal sex.

Taking Off the Gloves

Avoid touching the outside of the glove you used to touch the anus with. To remove your gloves, put a clean finger under the cuff of the glove and pull it down and right off your hand at once, so that the glove turns completely inside out. This way you won't come in contact with any part of the outside surface of the glove. If both hands are gloved, wash your hands carefully after removing your gloves.

Cleaning Sex Toys and Lube Bottles

Again, if you touched your bottle of lubricant with a gloved hand that had been inside the anus, wash the outside of the bottle off carefully as well. Try to avoid touching the cap with the same hand you are using to touch the anus with as the cap is often a harder part of the bottle to get clean. The easiest way to keep anal sex toys clean is to put a new condom on the toy each time. If you have silicone anal toys, you can boil them in water for 2 to 5 minutes. Remember to wash your hands after cleaning toys and lube bottles.

Chapter 10

There Should Be No Discomfort or Pain During Anal Sex

I must also say that there should not be any pain during any kind of sex for that matter. So, if you are having problems with pain during sex due to some kind of a physical ailment, then please give it the proper attention. Anal sex must not be painful! If you or your wife are to really enjoy it as a part of your love making. More to the point, you actually feeling pain means something is not right. (Please *note I'm talking about a sharp harmful pain not a full burning feeling that you WILL feel when you are being penetrated,)*

When the anus is really relaxed, it will admit a finger and even a hard penis quite easily. For sure it's a fact that both the internal and external anal muscles will relax and allow penetration, even if the natural design of the body is for one-way traffic. So, if there is some pain, just simply take a pause to work out what is going wrong. Maybe she is not lubed enough. Or maybe she has a fissure. Try to ensure that the receptive or passive partner knows they can stop your anal lovemaking at any point by using a safe word like "STOP" or "WAIT" if things get too distressing for them.

So, to avoid any discomfort, take it painfully slowly, and in the initial penetration which is where most of the pain is, ensure the wife can relax and open up for you as you move your finger or penis gently inside her. Bear in mind my friend, that the lining of the rectum is pretty sensitive. And it is much thinner than the muscular walls of the vagina. So, if you enter the anus with a finger, use the tender soft fleshy part to massage inside your lover's body, and also be sure you have trimmed your nails! Better yet use a gloved hand with plenty of lube on it.

Finger Penetration - The First Step to Anal Intercourse

Okay, if you want to penetrate them with a finger, simply use latex gloves for hygiene and sensitivity. If these things really bother you, just have some wet wipes ready to clean up. that way if there is any poop on your finger when you come out you can wipe it off quickly. Or use a small douche bag a few hours before enjoying anal pleasure with your man, as I have described already.

A cloth is useful anyway since you may want to wipe up excess lube which you have used to massage your partner's anus with, and liberally spread it over your finger or penis before you start your play. *(Lube your penis when you get to the stage of trying anal penetration with your cock)*. Now, you may be wondering just how do you penetrate the anus?

As we have already said there are two muscles rings around the anal canal, one on the outside of the body and one inside *(the internal and external sphincters)* They must somehow be tricked into opening up for you.

The anal canal is, of course, the very short passage that connects your anus to your rectum. These two sphincters are only about a half inch or so apart, but you both of them need to be relaxed before you can enter the rectum. And they can - as you may already know - clamp tightly shut. The external muscle will relax more easily than the internal one, which often clamps shut if you are feeling anxious or fearful about penetration. This is why it is so important you develop a physical and mental relaxation technique to trick the internal muscle. This is the key to successful, painless anal sex. The best way for anyone to do this is to insert a finger into their lover's anus and get them used to a finger being in there. Over time and continual practice, the muscle will stop being so worried about the intrusion from the outside. Quite frankly the more you do it the less pain is experienced. From experience of being penetrated by my wife's dildos, I know that the only pain that comes is a slight burning sensation like you have when you have a bowel movement.

When your partner is getting aroused, then you can begin to gently probe their anal opening with a fingertip. Bear in mind that you should have already lubed up everything really good before you start. Make sure you ask your partner if they are enjoying it, and if they are, and is okay with what you are doing as you progress. Opening up for anal penetration can be a very intimate act, so respect the fact that you are being given the opportunity to enter someone's body in this way.

Stroke and massage around their anal opening, giving your partner time to relax into the feelings of pleasure. When you both are ready, find the center of the anus and press gently into it with just your fingertip. As your partner relaxes and allows your finger into their body their pleasure will begin. This is usually best done as a conscious choice, that is an act of decision they have made with you to allow your finger to enter her. In other words, don't surprise her with a sharp poke. You may wish to gently move your finger back and forth. You should quickly find that your finger goes further into your lover's body each time you do it until it easily slides through into their rectum.

Okay, I'm inside my spouses' anus!

What do I do now?

Well, let's look at this from two points of view:

73

Man, Inside a Woman

Go ahead and bend down and use your tongue to stimulate her clitoris and vulva at the same time as you gently massage her G spot and other sensitive areas inside her vagina with one finger. At the same time, go ahead and play with her anus, her anal canal and then gently on the wall of her rectum with another of your fingers. If you massage the wall of her rectum closest to her vagina, you may actually find that you can convey exciting feelings through it, to her vagina. Of course, we need to re-emphasize the warning not to put a finger that has been up her anus into her vagina.

Woman Inside a Man

Well, the best thing I know that a woman can do for a man to simply massage his prostate gland. This can produce very exquisite sensations, though it may take a man a few sessions of anal penetration to get used to the idea and actually enjoy the sensations. *(This is rather like the way women have to get used to the sensation of having their G spot massaged.)*

If a man is lying on his back, with his legs up, which is the best way to massage his prostate. Just hook a finger slightly upwards inside him when you have penetrated his anus. Just softly massage it with a fingertip. Be careful, though, because the exact amount of pressure you need to use to give a man maximum pleasure is something that you can only establish by experience with him. So, start gently and work your way up to a harder push as he expresses his erotic pleasure. Try different movements of your fingertip. That is small circles, strokes, pressure, just be adventurous, and enjoy what you are doing with the man you love!

A male sacred spot massage is something your man will want you to try which you are doing it. It is all about the massaging of the prostate gland through the wall of the rectum. It can produce some greatly extended feelings of sexual pleasure and massive rolling orgasms without any ejaculation of cum in some men. If you're into this, try massaging different spots on the wall of his rectum and see how it feels, that is with or without an erection. Move your finger over as large an area of the rectal wall as you can until you've located the best spot for him. Moans of sexual pleasure are a good clue that you've found the right spot!

As you may know, much of the semen that a man produces is made in his prostate gland. When you tenderly massage your man's prostate, you will encourage and increase the production of more of his semen. This will in turn add greatly to the power and force of his eventual ejaculation of cum. A man's ejaculate may at times taste different and be much runnier after he receives a prostate massage. So, with that being said, it may make oral sex to orgasm *(with a finger on the man's prostate at the same time)* a more pleasant experience, perhaps enabling you to swallow his semen if you normally find the taste a little unpleasant.

Chapter 11

What Is an Anal Orgasm & How to Give One!

The anal orgasm is, as you have already probably figured out, is an amazing orgasm brought on by anal stimulation alone. This actually means using an inserted finger, penis, or a sex toy to bring out the orgasm. All women are able to achieve it, but only a few have the ability to actually experience it with extreme pleasure. The sexual climax can be either complete or incomplete, depending on your ability to touch, and thrust into her at the right moment. Some lucky ones may come to experience an anal orgasm without even stimulating the anus, but by stimulation of the buttocks and anal cleft with just the tongue.

Most people do not really understand how it actually happens. Typically, through stimulation of the upper wall in the vagina or the G-Spot, through the wall shared between the vagina and the rectum. Yes, it's an indirect stimulation. But perhaps that's probably why so many women (and men!) praise its intensity. As a matter in fact, there is lots of evidence that suggests that some women that experience anal orgasm is qualitatively different from clitoral or vaginal orgasm.

So yes, as you will see anal orgasm is not just a 'convenient' theory trumped up by horny men who want to get their respective wives to try it. It's very real, and it's happening every day, and it can be taught how to do it painlessly. There are probably three main different sources of sexual stimulation that is produced by anal intercourse. The sensation from the anus, the rectum, and the G spot. Each of these tissues sends different sensory signals to the brain through different pairs of nerves. The anus through the pudenda nerves, the rectum through the pelvic nerves, and the infamous G spot through the hypogastria nerves.

The anal orgasm is thus achieved and described as a 'deeper' and more intense, longer lasting, and associated with greater feelings of ecstasy.

How to Give an Orgasm During Anal Sex

Sometimes it is really good to first start with a firm/soft massage of her buttocks. Try to use contradictory moves, to enhance her pleasure. That is using light vs. firm, teasing vs. real pinching, etc.

After firmly separating her buttocks just a little bit, start tenderly massaging the area near the anus, but this time use much gentler moves. With a well lubed finger you can start by circling the anal opening with extremely light moves. Once you insert a whole finger or your hard penis and you reach the rectum, there is another set of pleasures that come into play. The outer portion of the rectum has several nerve endings. The inner portion responds mostly to pressure.

When you feel that she's finally ready to cum, you will want to give her additional manual stimulation on the clitoris. Also, for women who really love a being stuffed full feeling, try simultaneous penetration of the anus and the vagina with a dildo. Carefully pairing it with light clitoral stimulation, as mentioned above. The intensity of the anal orgasm can be achieved by psychological aspects as well as physical ones. The anal taboo also adds to the thrill of the forbidden. The typical and most common myth against anal sex is that *(it's dirty!)* sometimes returns as a source of extreme excitement. Other people for some reason regard the anus as a secret, and special place. So willingly sharing it with a spouse is an act of openness and lovingly giving it away.

On the flip side, the easiest way to not have an anal orgasm is to become really determined to have one. Seeking it will for some reason create new pressures and disrupt the pleasure. Friend whatever you do don't actually try too hard and it will happen for you. Remember it is actually supposed to be pleasurable.

Your diet can also contribute to the erotic feeling of extreme anal pleasure. Having regular bowel movements and a sufficient amount of fiber in the system will sometimes prevent irritation of the bowel tissues, which then causes discomfort and ads up to muscular tension.

If you do it regularly, it will become easier. The more often you do have anal sex the more you will like it. Start doing it about once or twice a week and with good practice you should get used to it.

Guys when you are taking her in the butt, please don't forget all about her tender genitals. You can easily stimulate her to orgasm with your hand while penetrating her butt. Just make regular gentle circles with your hand around her clitoris. If she says it's enough, it's enough, because at one point it may start to swell terribly for her.

Sir, you may want to ask her to put a latex glove on her finger, lubricate it really good and insert it in your butt. See how you'll like it. It's almost guaranteed you'll moan the first time she does it.

Also, don't forget about woman-on-top position in anal sex. Try to include it in your lovemaking pattern every once in a while, when you are starting out.

Chapter 12

How Can I Make Anal Lovemaking Better For My Wife?

These are the Important steps that I took to start this great experience with Anal Sex with my wife.

When a woman gives in to anal penetration it is something that she does to make her man happy, right? They don't actually enjoy it, right? Wrong! Lots of women really enjoy anal play. *(And my wife is one of them)* The anus is actually extremely sensitive and when stimulated the right way, can lead to her having intense and really explosive orgasms! Many women also enjoy anal play during sex and oral sex, and lots of girls like straight up anal sex and even double penetration with a dildo as well. However, there are a lot of guys who don't know how to make it comfortable for a woman, so she can't really enjoy it. *(That's what this book is for)* If a guy doesn't warm her up enough or use enough lube when engaging in anal play, it's not going to be much fun at all for her. In fact, it will actually be incredibly painful for her! Here's how you can make anal sex something she really loves.

Use Enough Lube

The main reason that most women don't enjoy anal sex is that it can hurt her, and it can hurt badly if it's not done correctly! One thing that can contribute to this extreme pain during anal sex is not having enough lube. Lots of good quality lube is so very important during this erotic activity because the anus does not lubricate itself the way the vagina does. Without this external lubrication, the anus can become very dry, and then the delicate tissues can tear and bleed. Don't be afraid to dump a whole bottle of lube on her butt if you have to – when it comes to this activity, you really can't use too much lube.

The best lube for anal sex if you are using a condom is a water-based lube, yes a silicone lube is thick and will last longer *(which is important for prolonged moisture)* but it is not as easy to rinse off as water based lube is. So, search for a good quality, gentle water-based lube that is made in a real thicker formula. Never ever use a desensitizing lube for anal sex! While this may make her more "comfortable" in the beginning, she won't be aware if the pain becomes too much for her. This can definitely lead to tears in her anus or bowel that may require immediate medical attention. Good water-based lube *(and plenty of it)* is all you need!

Use Small Toys First

Anal Play Christians Can Like It Too

Most guys get really excited at the prospect of trying anal sex with their wives. They are eager to put their penises in that tight hole right away. However, unless you're a *really* small guy, you may be too big for her if she hasn't tried anything else before or been properly warmed up before. Even with lube, if she's not practiced at taking something as large as your penis into her anus, you're going to have to start with something smaller like a small butt plug or finger and work your way up to a penis.

Yea guys fingering the anus is a good starting point, since you can use one finger and then gradually increase to two or maybe even three fingers once she becomes more comfortable with it. But in my opinion small butt plugs can be used to get her used to anal stimulation during sex. We started out fingered first and graduated to a graduating three-piece butt plug set. Once she was taking the big one regularly, she was ready for my penis. And this seemed to work best for us since she was sometimes having a climax with them being inserted in her. Even if you're chomping at the bit to get it on with her backdoor, she's going to love it a lot more if you don't bombard her right away with something huge at first, like your penis. She will also be more receptive to have anal sex more often if it does not hurt!

Give Her Encouragement

Women also love to know that they're giving their men real pleasure – and they want to hear about it firsthand from you.

While she's having anal sex with you, don't be too shy to let her know how much you enjoy it. Let it all out right then– moan, grunt and gasp so she knows that your pleasure is genuine! You can also give her a few words of encouragement as you're warming her up with your fingers. Let her know how hot her butt is and how naughty and sexy she is for her doing this with you. She will absolutely love hearing how much you are enjoying it!

So, what, it's a little poop. This is a huge reason that most women don't enjoy having anal sex with their partners. *(And you will deal with poop from time to time, trust me)* They're afraid or embarrassed to make a mess in front of, or on you. This may keep her from ever having anal sex with you at all. She could be extremely apprehensive about fecal matter coming out of her butt during sex and she may think you'll laugh at her or criticize her for it. Let her know up front that you know it might get dirty – and that it doesn't bother you in the least. And if it happens – please don't freak out.

Simply, have a warm, wet washcloth nearby for clean up and take care of it as soon as you notice it. If you can, don't even mention it to her. You can also ease her fears about making a mess during anal sex by encouraging her to have a bowel movement first or maybe to do an enema first a couple hours before your play. Some women even find the enema process quite pleasurable.

Make Sure She's Aroused First

Friend, if she is not aroused, she's not going to enjoy anal sex with you, period. Her anus will be too tight and puckered, and it will not relax enough to allow you to put anything in it, including your penis. So, before you plan on heading to her backyard for some play, play in the front yard a little first. Give her some great oral sex first and get her really, really turned on.

Carefully lick her clitoris and get her to where she's actually begging you to finish her off. Then, proceed to warm her up anally and don't neglect her clitoris when you do get started back there. With a combination of clitoral, anal, and even vaginal or G-spot stimulation, you may end up giving her the best climax of her life!

Take Care of Her Afterwards

When you are finished friend, listen to me for this is very important. Do not just roll over and go to sleep, even if you're really tired and tempted to. Instead, try to have a conversation with her. Help her get cleaned up with a warm cloth or join her in the shower if that's what she wants to do afterwards. Let her know how much you enjoyed it and how glad you are that she did it with you. Let her know that you care about her and show her that you don't think any less of her. Show her that she is very important to you and try your best to fulfill her emotionally as well.

If you do succeed and make her, feel good emotionally after having anal sex, she will definitely want to have it again with you. At the end, immediately following her climax, she may also become extremely sensitive to any kind of penetration. Thrusting or pulling out should only be done very gently after her orgasm. Also, you must remember that once your hard penis has been inside her rectum, don't put it inside her anywhere else.

Anal sex is one of the most erotic and satisfying sexual practices you and your lover can enjoy. It may take some time to get it just right, so remember you will both have lots of fun trying. The most important aspect of anal sex is good communication. So be sure to talk to your lover about your anal desires before, during, and after your first session of anal sex. I'm sure you're reading this because you really want to make your sex life exciting. You want to make it hot, passionate, and mind-blowing for her and you also probably want to find ways to please her. So, if you are ready to add more heat to the bedroom, keep reading my friend.

Sex Toys for Men

Though many sex toys are sadly depicted to be primarily for use on females, male toys do exist as well. These include things like cock rings, butt plugs, anal beads, artificial vaginas, and of course male masturbators.

Cock Rings

These are either made of leather or simple rubber rings that simply fit over an erect penis. The main reason people purchase these items is the help the man keep his erection for a longer time span. Many people swear by them though others feel that it doesn't keep them erect any longer. Two types of cock rings do exist: ones which are adjustable and ones which cannot be adjusted. If you are going to try one for the first time, go with one that can be adjusted for your penis first.

Multiple Sized Butt Plugs

These unique little toys are specifically designed for anal play. Butt plugs are carefully inserted into the anus for increase stimulation of the anus, which many males as well as females do enjoy. There are many men who enjoy this because it also stimulates their prostate gland. Butt plugs have many designs and are made with many different types of materials and colors. Some even vibrate after they are inserted.

Graduated Anal Beads

Anal beads are simply beads that are attached to a string and usually have a ring on the end where you can stick your finger through to control it. Using plenty of lube, you can then insert each bead in the anus one at a time and they are removed during sex play or orgasm. You can also take the anal beads out during two different times. Many pull each bead out one at a time slowly during orgasm while some people take each bead out during random sexual events such as during a rear entry (doggie style) position or during oral sex.

Climax Beads

Beads are some of the most popular of all anal toys. They range from really soft to firm-textured, and usually consist of four up to ten rubber balls connected with a piece of nylon cord or plastic/rubber. There is a wide selection in ball sizes graduating for small to larger. Whichever type you are interested in, they are virtually the best toys to ease into anal play.

Climax beads are a very simple toy to use. After being covered with plenty of anal lubricant, they are inserted into the anus slowly bead by bead from small to larger. Most people then leave the beads where they are until near the point of orgasm, at which time the beads are pulled out one by one. This can greatly intensify an orgasm to the point that it is too intense to handle.

Anal Play Christians Can Like It Too

We suggest starting with smaller balls, for they will stretch her out so she can then move up to larger, as you get more experienced. And like everything else that is involved with anal play, cleanliness is of the highest importance. Make sure to clean your toy thoroughly after using it, with alcohol and store it in a dry dust free place, and be very gentle when starting out.

Chapter 13

Relaxation Techniques For The Person Receiving Anal sex / Anal Stimulation

You must learn to relax your anal muscles. A great practice to use to learn how to relax your anal muscles is by trying to tighten them. Just clamp down on your anal muscles as hard as you can and hold for about two minutes. Then stop. By default, your anus is now relaxed. Once you have identified and learn to relax your anal muscles, try relaxing them without first tightening them.

Visualize positive sensations.

You must remind yourself often that you are engaging in anal play by choice. Your partner wants to please you with this special gift that they can give you. She/he is having fun exploring your body and watching your reactions. *Slow your whole body down by simply taking deep slow breaths. Don't do it if you're constipated.* Act like she is in childbirth and talk your lover through the breathing exercises. Make sure you tell your her that there are no time pressures at all. The goal is to only move forward when both people are ready to move forward.

You can also tell when your lover has totally relaxed his / her anal muscles, because they will feel relaxed to your touch. From a technical perspective, as we have already said several times there are two muscle rings surrounding the anal opening, otherwise known as the sphincters. One sphincter is involuntarily controlled by the central nervous system and the other is controlled by you and your central nervous system. The external sphincter is the one that you can learn to relax very simply. The internal one is automatic, much like blinking your eyes is. To locate these sphincters, just put your finger inside the anus and insert it a half an inch or so. As you touch the walls, you should be able to feel the two different muscles. They are located very closely together.

Talk Dirty / Sexy To Them

Try to use very positive images. Distract your lover's brain from focusing on the 'dirty' parts of anal play, such as the fact that you will get poop on your fingers. Use erotic language to direct your partner's mind to visualize his/her mind on the sensations.

Tell your wife that it is okay if they feel the need to poop. Your goal is to help them relax in the new sensations she is feeling. If your wife is so worried about the full feeling, they may tighten up too much and have difficulty relaxing.

As you intentionally move closer to the anus, ask your her if it feels, okay? Ask her for permission to keep going. Sometimes lovers do need an extra few minutes to catch his or her breath.

To penetrate the anus, start with your small finger. Cut your fingernails. You do not want to tear the lining of the anus. Then use a lot of lubricant. Never forget there is no such thing as too much lubricant. Start with using a steady slow touch. Insert your finger in straight. Pull it out slowly. Repeat. Go slowly. As you move about, tell your wife what you are about to do, so that he/she is mentally prepared.

Ask your wife to practice tightening and relaxing his/her anal muscles. Continue using one finger. Move your finger in a slow circle inside the anus. Again, ask your her for feedback. What type of touch feels most pleasurable to him/her?

In the beginning just five minutes of anal stimulation may be more than sufficient to loosen her up. Getting comfortable with anal stimulation or anal love may take weeks or even months. The truth is sometimes a person never does get used to it. Each of us is unique and experience things differently. Your job is simply to get to know your partner better and to help him/her get the most out of this very pleasurable sex act.

Once you are finally able to use one finger on five different occasions of anal play, then try using two fingers. Before engaging in penal anal sex, make sure you help 'warm up' your partner's anus by using your fingers first. Then upon initial penetration. The person receiving anal sex can then be in control of the speed of the penetration. Anal sex can also be pleasurable either from the mental perspective or from the physical perspectives. Ask your partner how they view it. Then get creative and build upon whatever their answers are. For example, if your partner is aroused from the dirtiness of anal sex, how then can you create a dirtier image for them to revel in? In contrast, if your partner is totally disgusted by the dirtiness of anal sex, but also truly enjoys the erotic sensations, how can you help your partner focus on just the pleasurable sensations?

Chapter 14

Anal Sex Positions

Your positions should only be limited by your physical ability to get in and out of them and by what feels comfortable for the both of you. Some positions will work out wonderfully for some and not for others. It's up to you to determine which ones work best for you as a couple.

Let me now give you a few suggestions to start with. Use this for a good first-time position. The first one and probably the most important one in my mind is with the woman on top facing away from the man. Sometimes called the reverse cowgirl. I say this simply because if it's your first time experiencing anal sex, this position will completely allow the woman to have control of the insertion of his penis into your butt.

This position is probably what most woman use for their first anal experience. It actually feels really comfortable because she has the control over how far his penis is going or not going to penetrate her with. She can stop when she feels she needs time to adjust to the full burning sensation and then continue when she feels ready to take on more of your penis.

This Is Still Many Women's All-time Favorite Position.

Ladies, all you need to do position is to straddle your husband facing away or towards him. Make sure that you've got lots of lubricant applied to his penis and to your butthole. You want to be able to have his penis slide in real smoothly. Just grasp his penis firmly and position the head at the opening of your anus. Hold it in place while you gently push your rear down against it. It will then move fairly smoothly for the first little bit and then you are going to encounter some resistance. this is where the muscular ring is.

To get past this point, you really need to relax and push down gently until you feel it pop past the tight muscle. Now, you might want to take a minute here to absorb how it feels so far. You may also feel like you're going to poop yourself. This is a very normal feeling, and trust me friend, you will not actually poop yourself. Some women also suggest that breathing plays a very big role in successful anal intercourse. It has been their experience that a woman will have a much easier time of it if she controls her breathing. If the woman takes a single deep breath and then exhales slowly during that first initial penetration it will also make the act more pleasurable for both partners.

Once you have adjusted to the full feeling, try pressing down further on his penis, taking more of it inside you. This is a really good time for your partner to play with your breasts, or stroke and play with your clit or whatever else works for turning you on. The more sexually excited you are the less attention you are going to pay to any discomfort that you might feel. Then you can start moving up and down on his penis, letting it slide in and out of your rear hole. You are in complete control and can also wiggle from side to side, move up and down as slow or as fast as you'd like. You can also control the depth and the force of penetration. When you're comfortable with this full feeling, you may allow your husband to become more of a participant instead of having him just lay still and remain passive. It's all up to you. I don't think that he's going to argue too much, especially if this is something that he's wanted to do for a long time and is finally getting the opportunity.

Sitting Anal Sex Positions

If a naked man simply sits on a chair or on the sofa, and his erected penis is pointing straight up, the lap dance can have an extremely erotic riding ending. While his partner facing a way, she can lower her anal opening down on to his penis, while she also supports herself with her arms, hold onto his legs. She then transfers some of her body weight to his legs from her butt.

How much weight she does depends on how hard she likes the penetration into her butt hole to be. She is the receiver, but she also controls everything. The depth, the speed, and the angle too. He just has to sit there and enjoy the amazing view... or he might just lie down on his back and feel really comfortable, because he has nothing to do. She is going to bang herself into an incredible anal orgasm. The man should just lie down on his back but he might want to prop up his back with pillows so he can see better. Of course, his penis should be hard like a rock and his wife should, sit on that rock-hard penis, facing his feet. She should grab his knees for support and ride him. He does not have to do anything, just sit there and let her ride. She is in total control. She can also control the penetration's deepness, the rhythm, and the speed too. If she wants to, she can ride him like a wild woman. If you have a toy like a high-speed miniature vibrator, she can use this on him between his anus and his balls. If he feels comfortable with it, she should then rub around his anus too. He will feel the vibration on his prostate gland, and he might also have the best orgasm ever. Also, his view is a sure mind blower too.

There are many more positions and techniques to try with your lover. Many people can also discover new and quite exciting positions through simple experimentation. And most people find the one that best suits them. Good communication is the key to such discovery. Regardless of you and your lover's sex life, or regardless of which sex position you try, the important thing is to use plenty of lubricant, and start slow, wait for the butthole to relax, and accommodate you. If you, do it right, you and your wife are going to feel sensations that you never felt before...

Most of the good anal sex positions are really just basic regular sex positions adapted a little bit for anal penetration. The two key factors for all good anal sex positions are that they also allow the receiver to be relaxed and physically comfortable and that it gives the person doing the penetrating available access to the whole anal area. Because anal sex is a much slower form of penetration, anal play is important to find a position that you're comfortable with and isn't too taxing on your body. Below are some of the most common anal sex positions.

Doggie Style

This the most popular rear entry position. Commonly known as doggie style *(My favorite)*. *It* is probably most associated with anal sex. This position gives easy access to the anus for penetration play, but because it doesn't allow for face-to-face positioning, it may be better for lovers who have experienced anal sex together and know what they already like.

If you are a nebbie at this and just beginning to explore anal penetration the side by side or knees on chest sex position might be better as it allows the wife to have more control, and more immediate non-verbal feedback about what's working and what isn't.

A position that really ,works so well for regular vaginal intercourse and also is a good choice for anal intercourse as well. Just simply kneel on your knees and elbows, remembering to relax your butthole. Your husband then kneels directly behind your butt, facing towards you. He will then bend forward guiding his penis to your anus opening as he gently pushes it inside. Entry is made easier if you try to draw his penis into your butthole as he is pushing. Push back against him as if you were trying to use the bathroom. As you relax with each push your anus will then slowly suck his penis into you. Your partner can then move his penis around inside your butthole by thrusting his hips forward and backward, while you either remain still or can move your hips from side to side. This position allows for fairly easy and allows for deep penetration.

Knees on Chest: Feet to Chest

The knees to the chest or other variations with the person being penetrated lying on their back with their legs up, can be a great first-time anal sex position as well. Both partner's bodies are close to the ground which allows for more relaxation and less work. It also allows for plenty of erotic physical touching which is so important during anal play to and it's easy for either partner to use a sex toy to add to more stimulation. Placing a pillow under the lower back of the partner being penetrated can also be helpful.

Now the absolutely easiest anal sex position, is known as the spoon sex position where both partners are simply facing the same direction. You can vary this position by having one partner almost on their knees penetrating the other partner who is lying on their side. The partner being penetrated can spread their legs in a scissor fashion. This position also allows for a great variety of angles of penetration without having to switch positions.

Side by Side Spooning

This position is just anal sex, with man lying on his side behind a woman. As we've said rear entry works very well for experienced lovers, but don't try this position the first time you have anal sex, because the woman is less in control in rear-entry positions.

This is a very good anal sex position, especially for couples who are for the first time just experimenting with this erotic activity. That is because when the man and woman lie on their sides, with the man behind the woman, it generally makes frantic thrusting quite difficult for him, which may put the woman more at ease.

Often the position that is recommended for people being penetrated for the first time *(whether it's anal or vaginal penetration)* that they start out on top. The benefit of the woman being on top is that she is in control of the rate of penetration.

Chapter 15

Analingus, Rimming/Risks (Known As Tossing Their Salad)

First of all, as I've already said in previous chapters; rimming is not necessarily a dirty exercise. The first thing you must get out of your mind is that the anus or butthole is dirty. It has been found through studies that most of the bacteria that is found around the anus are not harmful to us. And the area around the anus has also been shown to contain much fewer bacteria than the human mouth. So, if licking your lovers butthole is still a problem for you all you have to do is just shower before anal play and use a dental dam to block the hole.

Second and probably the most important is the "First Touch." Once you have overcome the reluctance of anal play, you then need to get used to being touched around this area. What you can do is simply get your partner and get some lube and get your lover to touch you around this area for fun. Have your lover run one finger between the cheeks of your buttocks. This may take some time and trust building. When both parties are really comfortable with this motion, you can then go one step further and press the pad of your thumb against their anus.

Analingus The Real True Love Kiss

This butt licking method is also be known as "analingus". It involves lots of kissing, licking, and sucking on the anus. For most people the primary fears of rimming have mainly to do with the smell, taste, and personal preference. If these things are a concern to you, then perhaps the ideal time for this sort of exploration would be right after getting out of the bath or shower. You can also buy dams as I said that are, made from latex, very similar to the dams they use in the dental offices, only a lot thinner. You would apply this to the area with a little lube to hod in place, so that your mouth would not be coming in direct contact with the person's butthole. But they would still get all the great sensations that come from being licked and penetrated by a tongue.

Analingus is amazing for the receiver and works so well because the anus opening is so incredibly sensitive. When the lips and tongue of your lover are warm and expressive it can really feel amazing. It's easy to do and can be done in any sex position where the buttocks can be spread far enough apart to admit the tongues entrance. Just run your tongue directly over the anus, tenderly licking it in soft wet strokes. Or circle it, by running your tongue all around the edge of it really slow and delicately. You can flick the tip of your tongue rapidly over the opening or try inserting your tongue as far as it will go by pushing and stroking it back and forth. Try brushing your lips over the spot or even sucking hard on the anus.

If you are the one being rimmed, try your best to push down the anus and relax the anus as if you were going to the bathroom. When you do it will expand a little outward giving your partner more area to caress or nibble at. It's best to just use your imagination and experiment with them a lot. But most important remember to pay close attention to your partner's reactions to all your different actions and techniques.

Why Do People Like Rimming or Being Rimmed?

Quite frankly I like this form of oral sex because it feels really great! Plus, I love to perform rimming to please my lover because she really loves it as well. I can actually feel her body melt under the pressure of my tongues entrance in her butthole.

The anus and all the outer area of the anus, that is the perineum, are highly sensitive and some people like this area to be touched, licked, kissed, tongued, nibbled on, or gently sucked. This is because this is an area that is full of dense nerves. Tongues feel moist and really warm and for most people having this area rimmed is highly pleasurable both, male and female alike.

Many people call this incredibly pleasurable sex an act a homosexuals and lesbians, but so are kissing and hand holding. Should we allow these perverse people to steal those sex acts from us too! Just like passionate kissing there are also many heterosexual married couples who perform the anal rimming sexual act on each other. If this is not for you fine. But don't condemn others that find it pleasurable and erotic.

Some Health Risks of Anal Rimming

The anal region will normally carry bacteria from the human body. There are some of the risks that are involved with anal rimming. Escherichia coli (E coli) can be transferred by a person who has just rimmed someone with it. When they go onto kiss their partner on the mouth and lips or even when giving fellatio (oral sex). In this example the E coli can be transferred down the urethra, where semen and pee come out and into the urinary tract and could at the least cause a urinary tract infection.

Other health hazards of rimming, especially if performed with no protection, are sexually transmitted diseases (STD's) like genital herpes, Gonorrhea, Human Papillomavirus (HPV), Hepatitis A, Hepatitis B, Hepatitis C and HIV (the virus that causes AIDS). Rimming can transmit giardia, amebiasis, shigella, and cryptosporidium. But since you are married you and your partner know each other well and especially if they are healthy everything should be okay.

How to Do Safe Sex Rimming

As we have said anal rimming is said to be a risky sexual activity, but so is kissing because there are more bacteria in the mouth than the butthole. The risks can be reduced by covering the anus with a plastic sheet called a dental dam which is available online. It is possible to buy flavored dental dams in flavors like cola, strawberry, and vanilla. A homemade dental dam can be made for anal rimming by cutting the bottom ring off of a condom and then splitting it up the middle so that a plastic sheet is made from it. An advantage of this method of safe sex rimming is that the rimmer can use flavored condoms to add some fruit flavor to the action. Another alternative for safe anal rimming is to use a ribbed condom for some extra excitement and more sensitivity. Some people even use latex examination gloves like those used by nurses and doctors. These can be bought at most supermarkets, by the cleaning or DIY products. If you do make sure your partner does not have a latex allergy and try to buy powder free gloves.

Another homemade protection for rimming is simply non-microwaveable plastic wrap. Though this may not offer as much protection as a dental dam. For sure the person who is receiving the rimming should give their anus a really good wash with warm soap and water before the sex act takes place. This will also reduce offensive smells and clingers but not reduce risks from blood if there are anal tears or cuts, hemorrhoids, or even fecal matter from analingus. It is normal to have light traces of fecal matter in the anal canal and this can be tasted or evident when giving analingus.

Some cautious people will use an enema before they do this sexual activity in an attempt to clear their bowel passage really good for their lover. This should be done several hours before sex to ensure the excess fluids are absorbed by the body and then expelled. Some people find that having an enema is uncomfortable whilst others find it very erotic. Regular use of enemas is not recommended though because it can disrupt the normal pattern of a person's bowel movements and could lead to bowel muscle wastage.

The recipient of rimming is also at health risks from their partner if he or she has some cold sores or open wounds in their mouth. Some anal rimmers may also like to use a mouthwash after they partake in rimming their lover. This is a sometimes-hopeful attempt to reduce the bacterial contamination and to hopefully reduce offensive smelling breath. The risk of catching Hepatitis from anal rimming can be greatly reduced by having a vaccination for Hep A or Hep B. This may be available at your local sexual health clinic or GP practice.

Special Analingus Techniques

When we are using the latex barriers during anal rimming put some lubricant under the dental dam or saran wrap barrier or improvised condom sheet to make the whole experience more comfortable and pleasurable for both partners. The person that is receiving the anal rimming should then kneel down into the doggy style position of being on their hands and knees. The rimmer can then gain better access to the anal passage by spreading their buttock cheeks apart. Doggie-style anal licking also provides quite a fantastic rear view, and allows you to squeeze, rub, and pull-on other areas as you lick away. Those receivers who have lower back pain or mobility issues can also simulate the doggie position by lying on their stomachs with pillows under their hips, comfortably raising their butts up for their lovers optimal licking. Another anal rimming position, but not for those with sore joints or back problems, is to stand and then bend at the waist to touch their toes or grasp their ankles. The one that is doing the rimming will then get behind them and squat or kneel down to give them a rim job.

A more comfortable rimming position is to lie on your back with a cushion or liberator ramp under your hips for support and to raise the anus up for easier access. Anal rimming can be an enjoyable sexual act between married couples and with a little preparation and care can be done safely and comfortably.

Some women get introduced to anal rimming when they are being eaten out by their man and an over enthusiastic tongue wildly reaches further down and gently strokes their anus or perineum.

Anal Rimming is something that you should discuss openly together before performing the act so that there are no sudden surprises!

Chapter 16

You Can Make The First Touch Of The Anus So Special

So here we go friends. With moistened softened lips, just kiss it directly. Then with the very tip of your tongue, lightly lick in a circle around the rim of the opening, "rimming" them.

Then lick the entire furrow with a big, flat tongue all the way from top to bottom like an ice cream cone.

You might then want to press your flattened tongue against the anal opening and just hold it there for a few seconds, before you slowly start to move it in an up and down or an in and out massage.

You can start with one of these techniques and try them all out to see what they really like. Since different people like different techniques, experiment with the ones that I have given you below to see which your partner enjoys the most.

Flicking: Gently flick the tip of the tongue across the outer rim of the anus.

Ringing the Bell: Push your tongue against the anus, and then quickly remove it, as though you were ringing a doorbell.

Licking: Use your full tongue to lick completely across the anus.

Probing: Insert the tongue as far into the anus as you can. Then simply probe around with the tip of your tongue. After a bit of gentle probing, both sphincter muscles should start to relax and welcome some deeper exploration.

The truth is many people won't orgasm by anal sex alone, so you should keep analingus fairly brief. *Most of the time, but not always I've ate my wife's butthole out for over an hour before with her going crazy the whole time.* You can also keep them stimulated in some other way at the same time.

Analingus is one of the most erotic intimate of all sexual acts a couple can participate in. If both partners approach it with openness and enthusiasm, they will be greatly rewarded with lots of unparalleled enjoyment. So, whether analingus is the main course, or just a spicy side dish, or an even appetizer for anal penetration. It is worth giving it a try.

If you do want to try analingus, but your partner doesn't, then by all means please don't try to force them! You have a much better chance that they will try it if you have their cooperation, rather than arguing with you. Bring the topic up gently on occasion and help them open up to this experience by getting them comfortable in the area and with the idea.

And always remember before you actually engage in analingus, make sure to thoroughly wash the area. A bath or a shower is a great primer and can be the start of the festivities. Once clean, licking this area of the body is virtually no different than licking any other, and can be very stimulating for both you and your partner.

Without going too close to their anus, explore their inner thighs and their bottom with your hands and mouth. Some people (*especially women*) have had bad experiences with anal play in their history, mostly because their partner moved much faster, or less gently, than they should have. If this is true in your case, getting them to talk about the topic is a great way to start. By learning where they went wrong, you can prevent that experience from happening again.

Chapter 17

Advance Analingus Techniques for Both Men and Women

So, listen to me ma'am, when giving your man analingus, there are a number of different things you can do to give him a lot of pleasure.

Up, Down & All Around

This is by far the easiest technique you can use for giving your man a rim job. To perform the Up, Down & All-Around technique you simply need to use a lot of saliva and keep your tongue loose and flexible. You simply need lick your man's anus up and down using your tongue or make a circular motion with it around and over his anus.

Just make sure that the entire time that you are doing this, that your tongue will be outside his body and on his anus. Remember to focus on mostly his anus, but also around it.

Poking Your Tongue Inside

After using the Up, Down & All Around for a few minutes, it's time to start moving on to more advanced rim job techniques like the Poking Inside. The Poking technique in simply as its name states. It requires you to make your tongue a little more pointed than usual and use it to try and penetrate his anus. You'll find that you will only be able to get about half an inch inside at most.

Kissy, Kissy

After you are at it for a few minutes of giving your man a rim job with your tongue, it will start to get tired. To give it some rest, simply start using your lips instead. Again, try to use a lot of saliva as it feels more enjoyable than dry kisses.

Toothy Time

I refrain from even mentioning this because using your teeth when giving your lover analingus is sometimes not a great idea. However, when it's done right, it feels fantastic. Remember, you do not want to cause your man pain, so no biting! Instead, you need to drag your teeth slowly and gently over his anus. Again, this is a great technique to use when your tongue gets tired. Just remember that you need to be very gentle. My wife drives me crazy when she nibbles down there.

The Gentle Scratch

While you are using your tongue on your man's anus, you can slowly and quite softly drag your hands over your man's butt cheeks, so that your nails are slowly and gently scratching them. This only provides a small amount of stimulation, but when coupled with your tongue techniques, it feels really nice for him.

Go Ahead Use Your Finger

Using your finger to perform the same moves as your tongue is yet another great technique to use so you can rest your tongue. Luckily, it's also stronger than your tongue, so you can insert it into his anus and use it to stimulate his prostate or other areas inside his butthole.

Chapter 18

More Analingus Positions

There are a few positions that you should use to actually make performing analingus on your man easy for yourself. These positions are designed so that he naturally spreads his bum for you so that you have easy access to his anus, without it feeling like you are being suffocated!

Doggie

This position most resembles doggie style. You just need your man to get on his hands and knees on the bed. To make it even easier, get him to lie on his chest while still on his knees so he is pushing his rear into the air. This position is the most comfortable for your man.

Grab Them Ankles Sir

Some older guys will find this rim job position a bit uncomfortable, but it can be very enjoyable if done correctly. Get your man to simply stand up and then bend over so that he is grabbing his ankles. It's fine for him to bend his knees to make it more comfortable.

Grab Them Ankles (Lying Down)

This analingus position is very similar to the regular Grab Them Ankles position we just mentioned. All your man needs to do is to lie down on his back while grabbing his ankles and holding them up. This will make it very easy for you to stroke his penis while rimming his butt at the same time. My wife and I like to use a behind the head sex sling to hold our legs up in the air and make it more comfortable while we are getting worked on by our lover.

Before You Perform Analingus On Him (Warning)

Now that you have read this detailed book on how to give analingus to your man, there is one thing to keep in mind before you perform analingus on your man…Some guys just don't like it…in fact a few actually hate it. So, you may find that it's best to discuss it first with your man before you actually perform it on him, otherwise he may get a bit of a shock if you suddenly start performing it without him knowing what you are doing first. Of course, gentlemen all these techniques can be used on her as well so study up!

Anal Prostate Stimulation Explained

Anal prostate stimulation is a very hot topic these days. It has also recently been featured in a lot of magazines marketed towards women as one of the hottest things to do in the bedroom to heat up your man. It has long been known that a simple finger in the butthole during fellatio will help the guy achieve a faster, more powerful orgasm. Recently, the popularity of these techniques has been surging. So just what is it, and why should you be willing to give it a try?

Ladies In this section, you will learn

The basics of anal prostate stimulation

Why prostate stimulation feels so good

Getting started with anal prostate stimulation

Understanding the basics of male anatomy will help greatly when learning about this technique. The male sex organs consist of three essential parts. The first, and the most obvious, is the penis. This is what is generally stimulated during intercourse. We all know that the testicles produce the sperm that comes out during ejaculation. Most people don't realize that the prostate gland is the third part in the male orgasm equation! This little gland is in the shape and size of a walnut and it produces semen, which is the fluid that combines with sperm during ejaculation. Most of his ejaculate is actually semen, and not sperm. This may be a shock to you, but it's really true! Stimulating the prostate is accomplished by reaching inside the anus. The prostate gland is protected by a thin amount of tissue on the top of the anus, about one half to two inches inside. This gentle stimulation will cause the prostate to go into overdrive, and it will produce more semen.

When stimulated properly, it will feel very good. This is because the majority of the good feelings you experience during orgasm first originate in the prostate gland. The combination of the increased pleasure will result in an orgasm that is very powerful. By applying a light pressure to the prostate during the orgasm, you can also stretch out the length of an orgasm to somewhere between thirty seconds to two minutes! I know friend it is mind blowing!

So, now that you know the basics of prostate stimulation and why it feels so good, what can you do to get started? Most gals will start out by using their finger only. This is okay, but it requires you to have some latex gloves on hand. Going to the drug store to purchase latex gloves and lube is definitely going to result in some weird looks. You can skip the gloves, but it isn't recommended. Maybe finger cots will be the thing for you, but we don't recommend that you use a bare finger. Just go ahead and lube up his butt, and slowly slip your finger in, and see what happens.

You will know as soon as you find his prostate gland, because even a light touch is enough to release a wave of pleasure that can be seen through his cock and balls twinging. The best way to really get started, though, is with an introductory level toy. These toys are available from a number of manufacturers. There are some vibrating toys that can really enhance the experience. My wife uses a vibrating graduated anal bead like vibrator on me and that is amazing.

If you are ready to move on to trying this out with your lover, then you just need to ask. The prospect of experiencing an increased orgasm is great for many people, and a lot of girls are willing to give it at least one try.

Chapter 19

The Benefits of Consistent Prostate Massage

This massaging effect upon the man's prostate creates a rhythmic pressure, and it is this gentle pressure that stimulates the prostate, resulting in the gland swelling and producing seminal fluid. Prostate Massagers simultaneously stimulates these zones to create intense, dry multiple orgasms.

Discover Prostate Massage Milking

The prostate gland is also composed of many tiny structures called acini, or sacs. Over time, if you lead an unhealthy or inactive lifestyle, the fluid inside can become stagnant or unhealthy. It's at this stage that bacteria can start to grow in these sacs. If that occurs, the acini can become inflamed and swell which can result in the acini sacs closing. This is a problem because it now means bacteria can build up without any way for it to disperse. The more acini cells that close themselves off, the more your prostate starts to swell, which leads to pain, sexual and urinary problems. The advantage of regular prostate massage milking is that is supplies the acini cells in the prostate with fresh new blood.

This in turn also enables you to thoroughly pass the accumulation of seminal fluid that has been collecting in the acini cells. Proper prostate massage milking also helps the prostate to rid itself of harmful bacteria so that the prostate can start to heal itself.

Another key benefit of prostate massage is that it also releases the seminal fluid that is trapped in your prostate without actually exercising the prostate muscles which are what cause ejaculation in the man. That emptying relieves you of the desire to ejaculate which occurs because pressure from the fluid inside your prostate gland makes you feel horny. Your body is basically saying it is full and wants you to have sex. That's great if you are prostate massage milking for sexual pleasure, you will undoubtedly feel a very pleasant orgasmic sensation from the procedure, but if you are trying to relieve the symptoms of prostatitis and you feel a real need for sexual release, prostate massage milking can help give your prostate gland both the release and the rest it needs. If you want to try your hand at prostate massage milking, the best way to do it is with an anal toy specially devised for the job.

The Secret to Prostate Massage

The prostate can also be a gold mine of sexual thrills for those willing to carefully probe and massage it. But while all the prostate sex manuals will tell you about the medical benefits to be enjoyed from prostate massage, it is also important to understand the risks.

The prostate is a very delicate gland responsible for the main production of seminal fluid. It's located just under the urinary bladder and is about the size of a walnut. It can actually be felt, and pressure applied to it through the lining of the rectal wall. As men age, the prostate can also become subject to a buildup of bacteria and can also be susceptible to cancer. This is why doctors will often check to see the prostate is not enlarged during a medical checkup.

When prostate massage is applied for sexual pleasure, the prostate then does swell and produces seminal fluid, which is an exciting sexual sensation. Indeed, with practice this can lead to the male multiple orgasm. The key to enjoying safe prostate massage is to go gently and never to rush. The new generation of sex toys such as the Aeros Helix or the Rude Boy are designed specifically to stimulate and massage the prostate safely without undue force being applied to the delicate membrane of the rectum. Correct use involves a medium to light repetitive massage or circular motion this tool is not intended for use in a thrusting manner.

It's also very important that you use plenty of water-based lube both on the sex toy and on the anus during prostate massage. If you feel any pain or discomfort during the session, cease and consider having a medical check up to ensure all is well.

Giving Proper Prostate Massage

If you mention to most men about the concept of having anything to do with anal play their reaction is not exactly encouraging. Anything that is remotely sexual that is connected to their anus has been taboo for hundreds of years. So even though giving prostate massage actually precedes the formal establishment of acceptable sexual practices and morals in medieval times. Generations of men have been taught that enjoying or practicing anal sex is bad, evil and you could even go to hell for thinking about it. It may even make you into a homosexual.

Now in these modern days they are being openly enticed to overcome these wrongful thoughts and beliefs to discover the joys of their partners giving them prostate massages. Unlike most everyday sexual practices that couples are involved in such as oral sex or simple sexual intercourse, giving a prostate massage does require a little understanding of the male anatomy. Pressure applied on this walnut sized gland through the membrane of the rectal wall can produce highly pleasurable sensations when giving the right kind of prostate massage. Push too hard or play too rough and it can be an uncomfortable, unsafe, and even dangerous procedure.

All that is required is some gentle downward pressure, either with a latex gloved finger, or best of all, with a specifically designed prostate massage sex toy such as the Aneros Helix, which hones in on the prostate. Also at the same time, massage the highly sensitive perineum, which is a cluster of nerves located between the anus and the testicles. Always use plenty of water-based lube applied either to the gloved finger or the sex toy when giving prostate massage. That's because the anus produces no lube of its own.

Powerful Orgasms From Prostate Massage

Assuming that you have already performed all the pre-session formalities we've talked about like urinating and having a good bowel movement, then by scrubbing yourself nice and clean, you are now ready to prepare for an intimate prostate massage orgasm. The prostate massage orgasm also can be done with a lubed latex glove, but the fingers actually fall a little short of providing the best orgasm.

If you are conducting prostate massage orgasm by yourself, first lube up your anal sex toy, because your anus produces no natural lube of its own, so it needs to be properly lubed. Also make sure there are no sharp edges on the device you use. Make sure is smooth all the way round. It should also be easy to disinfect after you use it. The best method of entry is to get down on all fours and slowly insert the toy - a sex toy is obviously safest and best because it is designed to massage the prostate and will not venture further up the rectum.

To insert simply inhale as you insert it in your anus. Breathing is also a very important part of a good prostate massage orgasm because you at the same time need to create oxygen for the nerves that you are massaging. As we have said the prostate gland is a sensitive organ located two inches inside towards the stomach. If you have already aroused yourself before starting, it will be easier to find the prostate because the prostate expands when it is pleasured. You can now start to add some gentle pressure along the wall of the rectum which starts to stimulate the prostate. Use a downward movement you will start to feel the powerful sensations.

As many men know a prostate massage orgasm can be a highly sensual experience which will blow you away and at the same time prevent a buildup of semen in the prostate gland. It's a cleansing and will improve the circulation and will actually make doing masturbation completely unnecessary for the man! Always massage gently and don't try it more than three times a week

Preparing for Prostate Massages

It's best first for you to urinate and/or have a bowel movement before you actually begin. Staying relaxed throughout the whole prostate massage is also very important. So, try to wind down first with a relaxing bath or shower before you start.

Another good way to actually start a prostate massage is to massage the prostate externally. Using the index and middle fingertips. You can then touch, rub, stroke, or press on the perineum *(the area of skin from underneath the testicles between the anus).* While you press on this center of nerve endings you can also stimulate other parts of his body so as to become more receptive for the actual prostate massage itself. If you opt for a sex toy such as the Aneros Helix, you will find this much easier and more convenient to use than fingers as it is specifically designed to locate the prostate and massage it cleanly and smoothly.

The Aneros can also work hands free, leaving you or your wife free to explore and arouse other parts of the body. The combined massage of the prostate and the perineum can provide highly intense sexual sensations, and can even produce a super orgasm, akin to the multiple orgasm enjoyed by females.

If you're using sex toys for prostate massages, always use a fresh condom on male anal toys, if you are exploring with your fingers, or your wife opts to massage you that way, use a fresh latex glove on the hands, and ensure that the nails are trimmed with no sharp edges.

It certainly can be a powerful fantasy and can be a deeply pleasurable experience, although you will need to bear in mind that anal sex isn't to every woman's taste, not by a long shot, and if the answer ends up being no, you're going to have to accept that. It's worth considering why you feel you couldn't actually ask your wife about anal sex. Is this because you know she'd say no? Is she a very conservative person, sexually speaking that is? Do you find it uncomfortable generally to talk about sex? If you can talk about sex in a relatively free and easy way, then you could work your way around to the subject of anal sex – to the point where you might feel able to pop this question. One very good way of broaching the subject would be to try different positions and read this book together. You can talk about and try out the many positions you see it can take a couple a good while to fully experience the real pleasure of anal play. This would give you the perfect opportunity to ask if your wife would like to try anal sex or if your husband is open to giving it a try – and you'll have expanded your repertoire in other new directions besides!

Another way of beginning to broach the subject is to offer some anal stimulation while giving your wife or husband oral sex. Gently caress their anus with a lubricated finger, or switch from oral to rimming them – and if they seem to like that you could suggest you try penetration. Of course, they might be wondering what the heck you're up to if you've never rimmed them before, but then you can say you got carried away, that you love their butt so much that you couldn't help yourself, right? Just kidding, but this might pave the way for more anal activity. Should your spouse decide that anal sex is something they'd like to try, and then you'll want to do as much as you can to make this a pleasurable experience for them especially for her! She might appreciate a more conventional orgasm first. Then use a lot of lube and a well-groomed finger to relax and open her up, and then penetrate slowly. Now, while you obviously want to see your penis sliding in and out of her butt, it can actually be more comfortable, on the receiving end, to adopt a deep missionary position, face to face with her legs up – and this can also be more emotionally reassuring. Hug and go slowly at first – those first thrusts set the tone for the experience to follow. You can always switch to a doggy sex position when you're both warmed up and ready to go guns. *(And don't then transfer your penis from her butt to her vagina, not without washing it thoroughly first.)*

When receiving anal sex, especially at first, it is normal to have the sensation that you're about to "go #2." The nerves in this area send that signal when they are triggered. This feeling will usually subside after a short period.

I pray that this book has aided you in your quest to have a safer more erotic experience in your marriage. Just remember that as a Christian we are called to do all to the glory of God so keep your sexual relationship with your spouse a God glorifying one and you will have a great life together. If you enjoyed this book, check out our complete line of Christian lovemaking manuals written by Kelly Walls. **Also leave us a review where you bought it that would be greatly apreciated.**

Kelly Walls

Copyright © 2018 by CLMS Publishing

Published by CLMS Publishing

Other Books By Kelly Walls

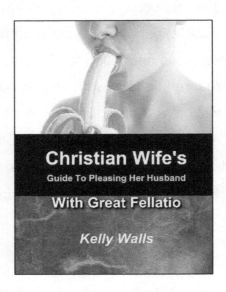

Does your husband arch his back and scream I'm cumming!

Today oral sex is like kissing if you aren't very good at it you won't please your mate to the fullest. That's precut probably because you had a bad teacher worse yet you had no teacher. Listen to me ma'am, don't be lazy and hone up your tongue skills and you'll never have to worry about losing your man. This book will teach you how to make your man so weak in the knees he'll actually want to pass out from pleasure.

In fact, my wife who is expert fellator has made me want to pass out at times. You will learn over 200 fellatio techniques that will make his eyes sink back in his head.

Many women approach the lovemaking act of fellatio with a sense of dread or obligation. Ladies this need not be so, as fellatio can - and should - be enjoyable for both the giver and the receiver.

This book will teach you how to take the job out of giving your husband a blow job. Fellatio is a great way to express your love and devotion to your man. Men find fellatio a lot more enjoyable as well when their wife is enthusiastic about doing it. Wanting to pleasure your man is often the best way to pleasure yourself, and blowjobs can be your ace in the bedroom.

So, do yourself a favor ma'am and give your man the greatest and most loving blowjob of his life. Keep reading to find out how. The problem is for so many people is that they have been trained by pornography. That is before they became a Christian. And pornography makes giving a blowjob look so easy. It seems you just put his penis in your mouth, and voila he goes off to orgasmville. However, sex in real life is much more complicated than that. Yet in real life it should be as enjoyable and intimate, then porn makes it out to be.

Now in days gone by the blow job was just considered a part of foreplay; but today in this modern day everyone knows it's a centerpiece of a really great sex life. But contrary to what most are saying not everyone who claims to be a deep throat expert really is one.

The art of sucking and licking your husband's penis has to be learned. In this book you will truly learn how to be a fellatio champion. You will learn about the secrets of deep throating and the caterpillar technique. A technique that will make him almost want to cum immediately.

You also learn what the Jade flute technique, is the harmonica technique, the cum thumb and the figure 8 and so many more.

Why gagging is such a powerful experience for your man; and why a powerful blow job can bring tears to your eyes.

This great guidebook answers these questions and many more. It contains over 200 Best Fellatio Techniques of fellatio fun.

You will learn how to make every time a new experience with your man. He will call you his blow job queen and his awesome succubus. Believe me he won't look at any other women.

Also, you might want to get your husband my new cunnilingus book or fingering book so that he'll learn how to blend bring more pressure to you.

Want to Learn How to Make This "Job" as Much Fun for You as It Is for Him?

Each page is laid out to give you several juicy tips on how to overcome the fear of going down on your lover.

Still not convinced, okay ladies, your man may or may not ask for it, but it's exactly what he wants believe me.

It's often his hidden, secret desire that you perform fellatio on him. Maybe's he's asked a time or two, but when that didn't work, he just stopped asking. Maybe he's one of the lucky ones and you give in and give him one on special occasions from time to time. But believe me after you learn how to do it right this will become so special to you that you will want to do it more. "Really ladies" if you want to pleasure your man and keep him home with you and not running around with the boys this is the key.

But if you really want to make your man, feel manly, confident, and wanted you'll fulfill this secret little dream of his. And he's going to be blown away (pardon the pun) when you give him exactly what he wants in a way that brings him the most intense pleasure. After you read this book, you'll have the confidence it takes to ensure a good time for the both of you... and your man will wonder what got into you.

Within its pages are loads of skills for satisfying your man along with tips on how to have a little fun for yourself along the way. You will learn how you can take charge in the bedroom, entering the bedroom with full confidence in performing oral sex and feeling like a champion while you're doing it!

Here is just a sample of what you'll learn:

- If oral sex is OK with God in the married relationship.
- The various ways to spice up your sex life with your man.
- How to communicate effectively with your husband by asking him some very specific questions.
- What your husband should eat to make things as pleasurable for you as possible.
- How to get started with sex toys IF you're looking for that something extra.
- How to make your husband squirm with pleasure and have him begging you for more.
- What to do with your eyes, hands, mouth, and tongue.
- How to practice with your tongue and a dildo till you become an expert.
- How to build anticipation and excitement in him.
- How to decide whether you should spit or swallow or do something else with his semen.

A woman that knows what she is doing while performing fellatio is able to connect with her man on a far deeper level. She can make her grown man moan, beg, and shake at his knees, all at the expense of the tricks she can perform with her mouth, tongue, and hands.

Fellatio for a man is the ultimate expression of love. Having the woman of his dreams caress his genitals to the point of an intimate, sensual, and mind-blowing ejaculation, is a feeling that is beyond words for any man to describe.

So, get a copy today and get ready Send your man to

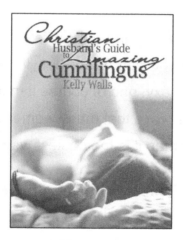

Heaven!

Are you giving your wife screaming orgasms?

If not you're like most guys that have no idea how to stimulate the clitoris. Is your wife shooting you in the face with so much cum you feel like you need goggles? Don't you dare settle for the lie that she is not a squirter! All women can squirt if they're stimulated correctly. So many men don't have a clue how to stimulate the clitoris. They finally find it and say to themselves; "there it is I guess I should rub it real hard." "WRONG!"

My friend there is a reason why it is protected by a hood and most of it is hidden except for the tip. It is because its only purpose is for her sexual pleasure. If you apply the principles in this book your wife will squirt you most of the time. She will scream with pleasure. She will wiggle all over the bed and grab your head and push it into her pussy and scream and call you a SEX God!

Listen to me guys, eating your wife's pussy is about the most wonderful thing you can do for her. It makes her feel specially loved, admired, sexy, and of course it makes her cum like crazy. In fact, statistics prove that many women prefer it to intercourse, and for most women it is the easiest way to cum with her man.

You may have the smallest penis on the planet, but if you give great cunnilingus, you will be appreciated as a fabulous lover. Yes, it's that important. Besides, lots of women expect it these days. So, you might as well know what you're doing.

Fellas, if you don't know it by now, know this. Cunnilingus is amazing to women! And all men must learn to respect the clitoris of their wife. It's a sex organ given to them by God Himself for only one function alone and that is to bring her pleasure. And with its more than 8,000 nerve endings, it does just that!

The main problem is that many men are reluctant to give their wife cunnilingus. Either they don't like to do it, they don't know how to do it, they don't do it often enough, or they don't do it long enough when they do-do it.

And worst yet of the guys that do give cunnilingus, not all of them know how to do it well. And most of them don't know how to set their wife at ease so she enjoys the experience to the fullest. Christian friends this book is your answer with more than 210 cunnilingus tips alone, you are sure to find something that will send your wife over the edge.

This book has been called the encyclopedia of the art of cunnilingus filled to the brim with over 100 pages of pure teaching on giving cunnilingus, vaginal and anal massaging, rimming and so much more. And if that was not enough it will give you a deeper understanding of the practice and help you and your honey have a better oral experience together.

And of course, as with all our books it is written from a Christian perspective taking into consideration what God has to say or has not to say about various topics. This I believe will help you take your cunnilingus skills to a new level.

Consider this sad fact guys. The average man who practices coital relations, that is thrusting into his wife's vagina lasts approximately 2 and a half to three minutes and the average woman take approximately fifteen to twenty minutes to reach her first orgasm.

So, what you do in the first twelve and a half minutes really makes the difference as to whether she will experience true pleasure at all. I fear that most woman end up finishing themselves off with their fingers after their husband is sleeping. This shouldn't be so in a vibrant healthy marriage. And most woman if they will admit it to you enjoy cunnilingus more that penetration from a penis.

Personally, I don't care if I get my wife off with my tongue, finger or penis as long as I get the job done and she enjoys the intimacy. As long as I leave her breathing hard and begging me to stop because she can't take it anymore, then I am pleased.

This book will teach you how to give her multiple orgasms with both your tongue and your fingers, also if you want a more detained guide on fingering and pleasing your wife with your hands get my book "Christian Husbands Guide to Fingering and Pleasuring His Wife with his Hands."

When you leave the bedroom, you will know that you pleased her and she will want to pleasure you with better fellatio too.

My friend most women want to reciprocate pleasure so you can get her my Fellatio book; "Christian Wife's Guide To Pleasuring Her Husband With Great Fellatio" for present and give it to her. It has over 200 fellatio techniques in it. **Get a copy today!**

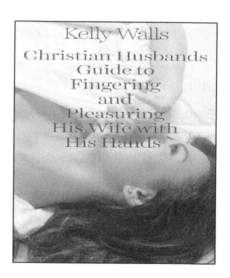

Is your wife screaming and squirting and begging you to stop because she can't take another orgasm?

If not, maybe the problem is you don't know how to use your fingers. You see sir the G spot is the pleasure center for the woman. And he clit was given to her by God for the sole purpose of orgasm. And to make matters worse most guys don't know how to touch it properly. They don't know how to stimulate it correctly. Most guys just sort of poke and rub all around hoping they do something that she likes. **If she isn't asking you to use your fingers on her then you don't know what you're doing!**

Another interesting fact is that most guys penises are shaped to stimulate the G spot, but they don't how to do it with them. Some men think they have to have a 10-inch penis to pleasure their wife. Not so my friend. I can show you how to do it and make her beg you for it with just your thumb. In fact, my wife prefers a thumb ride as she playfully calls it over any other kind of way to pleasure her sexually.

I'll show you how to make circles with your fingers that will make her squirt and scream at the same time. You will learn dozens of finger techniques to masturbate your wife with and stimulate her G spot with.

I promise if you use these techniques rubbed against the G-spot you will cause her to squirt at least half the time. She will go wild in bed and want to pleasure you as well. You might want to get her my new hand job secrets book that's filled with masturbation techniques that she can use on you to pleasure you as well. And believe me she wants to pleasure you.

The techniques you will learn will make you have to put a towel on your bed before you make love to her with your fingers.

Okay gents you want to learn more about pleasuring your wife with your hands that's why you are buying this book.

This book is a definitive guide to the female vagina and inside this guide you'll learn...

- step-by-step, techniques on how to finger your wife the proper way that will give her a mind-blowing orgasm.
- How to stroke her clitoris to produce clitoral orgasms and multiple orgasms are usually common.
- How to combine oral sex and fingering techniques.
- The best positions to finger your wife in during sex that will make her reach climax every time and not just about 40% of the time.
- Step-by-step instructions on how to find the G-Spot and what to do once you find it. Even how to play with her anus if she wants you too.

Guys this is the key to making her squirt you in the face with a squirting orgasm. Even if she has never squirted before these techniques will teach her how to get her to squirt with pleasure.

Anal fingering and massaging and the amazing pleasure that comes from this practice.

Dozens of techniques and strategies that will lead your wife to orgasmic bliss. A great buy! **So, get a copy today and have some fun! Buy a copy now!**

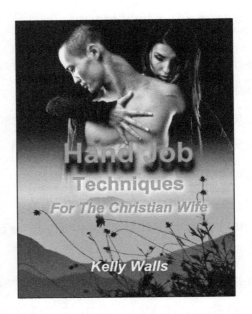

What most women don't understand is that men love hand jobs.

That's why they masturbate so much. In fact, some studies have shown that some men prefer them to fellatio. Go figure.

The fact is that pleasuring your husband with well-oiled hands rubbing and squeezing and pulling and sliding on various spots of the penis feels amazing.

So, ladies are you looking for new ways to spice up your boring sex life? Have you tried giving your husband a hand job only to discover it can be very tiring and boring?

If so, this book will teach you new techniques *(Over 70 masturbate your man techniques)* that will allow you to become an expert in pleasuring your lover with your hands.

With over seventy different moves called "masturbating him' you will definitely find the ones that please you both.

This book is designed to be a guide to help you learn and experiment with things that you probably never thought of before.

By all means masturbating your man is more than grabbing his penis and pulling up and down on it. It's more than jerking him off just the way fellatio is more than bobbing your head up and down.

This book will teach you the art form of pleasuring your man with your hands.

It includes descriptive explanations of the main techniques and extra useful information.

You will learn:

- The anatomy of a man's penis.
- Different types of lubes: A wide variety of hand job techniques:
- Basic, rubbing, twisting, sliding and so many more bonus techniques, guaranteed to give your man the ultimate pleasure.

Forget about awkwardness when giving a hand job! Open yourself up to a new and exciting experience in the bedroom and blow your lover's mind!

Ready to learn more? Pages and pages of raw loving making experience with just your hands, or feet, or breasts. Oh yes, we will discuss these methods too. **Get a copy today!**

Made in the USA
Las Vegas, NV
03 October 2024

96242484R00085